The 5-Ingredient
Low-FODMAP Diet
Cookbook

Affordable and Delectable Recipes to Soothe Your Gut, Manage IBS
and Other Digestive Disorders

By Katie Evans

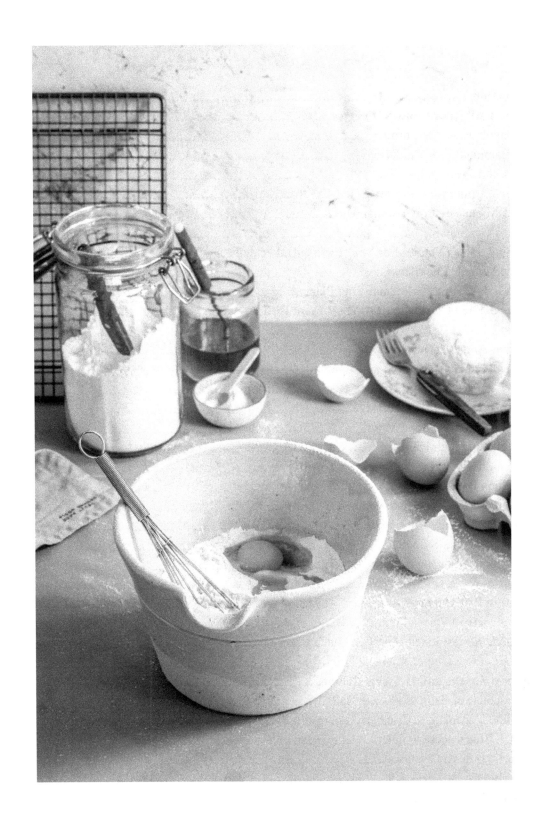

Table of Content

Introduction

As a registered dietician, I know all too well how the food we eat can affect our health in so many ways. If you suffer from gut-related health issues, then life can be miserable. It doesn't take a genius to conclude that changing what goes into our digestive system can significantly affect the symptoms and the severity of those issues.

IBS & IBD are miserable conditions. It can affect all aspects of your life. You may avoid socializing; it can affect your mood, sleep, confidence, and self-esteem in addition to uncomfortable and painful symptoms.

If you like up to 14% of Americans have a gut-related condition, then I have great news for you. By following a low FODMAP plan, you could be feeling better in 2 weeks or less! The best part of my job is restoring a person's health. Some diets can be a real hardship and difficult to stick to - they can also take a long time to have results. So often, the sacrifice can outweigh the benefits.

But that's not the case with a low FODMAP diet intended to reduce the symptoms of IBS significantly. When you suffer from IBS, you know when your symptoms have gotten worse or better. But it can be real detective work to pinpoint which food triggered it.

For instance, you might have a meal of Spaghetti Bolognese and Garlic Bread with a dressed salad and find yourself with terrible symptoms the day after. But what caused the problem? Well, that meal consisted of meat, vegetables, salad, pasta, bread, and cheese on your pasta. So, you have no idea what was the cause of your misery.

With a low FODMAP diet, you'll eat my delicious recipes that eliminate all the foods that could be causing your gut to react. And trust me, you won't feel like you're on a diet. For so many high FODMAP foods, there are low FODMAP foods that you can swap, and you won't feel like you're missing out.

It should be noted that my recipes are healthy, but they are not intended for weight loss. That being said, IBS can cause uncomfortable gassy bloating. And if you suffer from bloating, you may find that if these particular symptoms improve, your clothes will feel looser. And you'll look and feel slimmer without "dieting" at all.

The recipes are not low-carb but instead have a healthy ratio of fat, protein, and carbohydrate. There is a full selection of recipes that includes pasta, chicken, meat, fish, and plenty of desserts for those with a sweet tooth.

Many people with IBS and other gut-related illnesses suffer in silence for years, but for many, the problems can be solved quite easily.

All the hard work and research has been conducted by scientists who have developed a low FODMAP diet at Monash University in New Zealand. With the help of these researchers, there is now a super-easy way for many people to get their symptoms under control. And start living life to the full again.

Before I was a dietician, I was a cook with a passion. I also love solving problems. With my smart recipe adaptions, I hope you'll find my recipes enjoyable and soon be on your way to finding a personal solution for your gut-related health issues.

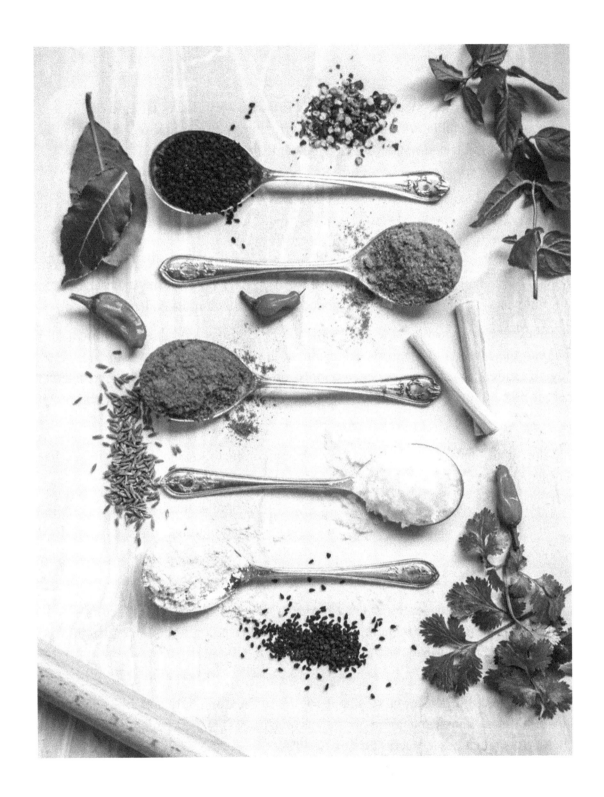

B oth Irritable Bowel Syndrome (IBS) and Inflammatory Bowel Disease (IBD) are painful and debilitating conditions. The symptoms can be the same, and often the outlook can seem bleak. First, let's take a look at them separately.

Irritable Bowel Syndrome

It's thought that as many as one in five Americans have IBS. The condition is more common among women, and symptoms vary in severity. The kinds of symptoms experienced range from flatulence, stomach bloating, and abdominal pain to diarrhea and constipation.

While for many people, the symptoms are mild, for others, they are present all the time, and they make life a misery. It's common in illnesses that cause pain and won't go away for sufferers also to experience depression and or anxiety. That's understandable. There is no cure for IBS. So that's a very depressing thing for your doctor to tell you.

Your doctor may have advised you to do some or all of the following things with or without success:

- Avoid spicy food
- Take exercise
- Cut back on caffeine
- Eat smaller meals
- Take probiotics
- Reduce stress

The other thing about IBS is that not only is there no known cure. Doctors still don't know what causes IBS. It's thought that an oversensitive colon or immune system may be the cause. Or a previous bacterial infection in the gut.

All of these things offer no real hope for the sufferer and only add to the anguish and despair. It's a real shame that more physicians aren't advising their patients to follow a low FODMAP diet that has a success rate of 75-80%.

Inflammatory Bowel Disease

IBD is an umbrella term for certain bowel diseases. It covers Crohn's Disease as well as ulcerative colitis. Just like IBS, the exact cause is unknown, but these are both severe illnesses.

Symptoms of IBD can also be similar to IBS with bloating, diarrhea, cramping, and stomach pain. However, there are far more severe complications associated with IBD. Patients with IBD can develop complications, including fistulas that go through the bowel wall, malnutrition, intestinal rupture, colon cancer, and bowel obstruction.

To diagnose IBD accurately, your physician may perform various tests. These include x-rays, barium enemas, endoscopies, colonoscopies, as well as blood and stool samples.

It's imperative if you have IBD, you minimize your risk of more severe complications. Make sure you eat healthily, drink lots of fluids, exercise regularly, and don't smoke.

IBS, IBD & Fodmaps

Both of these conditions are triggered by foods that are high in FODMAPs. It may be that you have undergone tests at the doctor's surgery. You've been poked, prodded, had your stools investigated as well as your blood. Your doctor may even have prescribed medication for you.

In studies, both IBS and IBD have responded well to a low FODMAP diet. But, you should not embark on a low FODMAP diet unless you have been diagnosed with either of the two conditions.

While the diet is safe, it's only recommended for those with digestive conditions. If you haven't responded to eliminating caffeine, alcohol, and spicy foods and other remedies suggested by your doctor, then you should consider giving this low FODMAP diet a go.

However, you absolutely must speak to your health professional before you do. The diet may seem a little complicated, but it's only a case of not eating the high FODMAP foods detailed in the FODMAP bible provided, and eating low FODMAP foods instead. Simple!

And you'll find 85 delicious recipes in the book to make. The recipes contain just five main ingredients. And most of the recipes are very quick and easy to make.

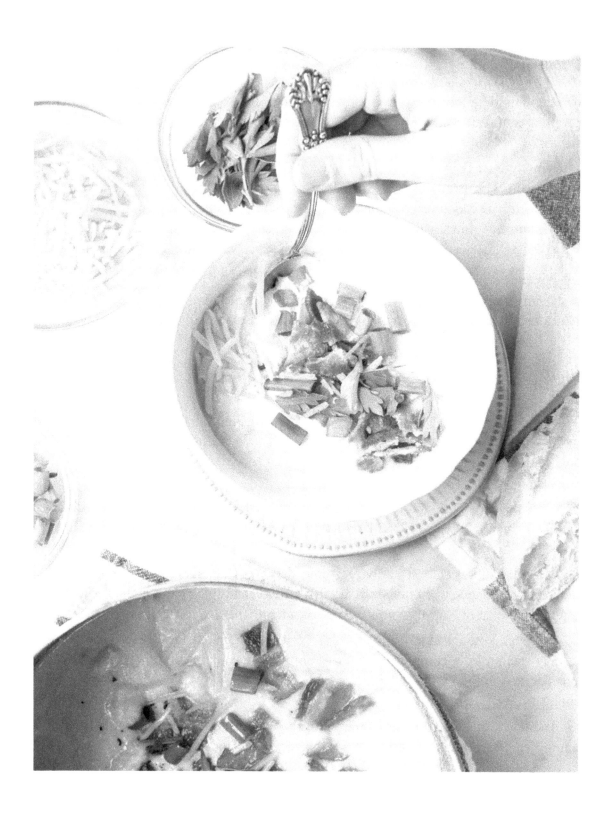

FODMAPs is an acronym short for:

- Ferment-able
- Oligo
- Di

- Mono-saccharides
- And
- Polyols

I guess when researchers first coined the term, they had quite a few choices. But it's not a bad choice. As learning about foods that have high and low fodmaps is a little like a map pointing you in the direction of better digestive health.

FODMAPs are types of carbohydrates found in certain foods, and they are linked to digestive symptoms in sensitive individuals.

Here Are the Main Types of Fodmaps:

Oligosaccharides: Carbs in this group include fructo-oligosaccharides and galacto-oligosaccharides. Found in wheat, rye, various fruits and vegetables, pulses, and legumes.

Disaccharides: Lactose is the primary carb in this group. Found in milk, yogurt, and soft cheese.

Monosaccharides: Fructose is the primary carb in this group. Found in some fruit, honey, and agave nectar.

Polyols: Carbs in this group include sorbitol, mannitol, and xylitol. Found in some fruits and vegetables, as well as many sweeteners.

FODMAPs are carbohydrates that are resistant to digestion are often classed as fiber. So any food that contains fiber may also be high in FODMAPs, whereas low and fiber-free foods are usually low or free of FODMAPs. Still, that's no excuse to stop eating fiber, which is good for us and in particular, bowel health. It's a case of getting clued up on FODMAP foods if you're sensitive to them and are struggling with digestive symptoms.

While most carbohydrates will have long since been broken down and absorbed into the bloodstream, FODMAPs are resistant to the digestive process and instead "survive" the long journey through your intestine and end up at the furthest end of your intestine where the gut bacteria is. The gut bacteria finally break down the FODMAPs producing hydrogen gas.

FODMAPs also have the effect of drawing liquid into the gut, often causing diarrhea.

Sensitivity to these carbs differs from person to person.

The low FODMAP diet developed by researchers from the Monash group in Christchurch, New Zealand, was aimed at helping people with digestive problems such as IBS and IBD.

The diet began development after 2004 when the term FODMAP was decided upon and has been a great success for many reasons. The diet is easy to follow and improves symptoms in around 75% of people with IBS.

IBS is not fully understood, but sufferers who follow this diet can expect to experience improvements in symptoms such as gas, bloating, stomach cramps, diarrhea, and constipation.

Not just that, because it's known that IBS can also cause stress, anxiety, and depression, followers of a low FODMAP diet may also see improvements in these symptoms too.

The diet can also have benefits for an umbrella of inflammatory bowel diseases (IBD), including Crohn's disease and ulcerative colitis.

The diet has also proved a great success because you don't have to wait long to see improvements. You may even be symptom-free in as little as two weeks and be ready to move on to the next part of the low FODMAP diet plan.

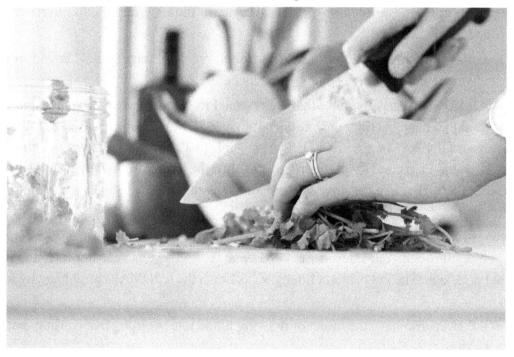

Let's Get Started

If you've decided that your symptoms warrant a change in diet and that you may benefit from targeting certain foods, then the best advice is to follow a low FODMAP diet for 2 to 6 weeks.

If your symptoms improve or disappear like in the case of 3 out of 4 people, then great news! If not, you should seek further advice from your medical practitioner.

There's no need to do tiresome research. Just stock your pantry and fridge with low FODMAP food and either follow our 4-week meal plan or select any of the low FODMAP recipes featured in the book.

Clear Out The Old And Start With The New

It's best to clear out your pantry of high FODMAP foods to begin the diet. And start over with low FODMAP foods. Use one cupboard for low FODMAP ingredients so that you don't add high FODMAP ingredients to your meals by mistake.

Low Fodmap Staples For Your Pantry and Fridge

Detailed here are a few basic food staples to stock your pantry and fridge with. You'll find a complete food bible in the next part of the book. There's also a list of ingredients to stock your store cupboard with if you intend to make my recipes.

You'll find a 4-week menu plan further on in the book. If you're going to follow this plan, then you can plan your shopping list of fresh ingredients for the week from this plan. Alternatively, read through the recipes in the book and draw up your weekly diet plan. You can then write a shopping list based on this plan.

Low Fodmap Staples For Your Pantry:

Oats, cornflakes, gluten-free pasta, rice, tinned tomatoes, chickpeas, gluten-free bread, rice cakes, sugar, gluten-free flour, quinoa flakes, garlic-infused oil

Low Fodmap Fruits And Vegetables:

Oranges, pineapple, kiwi, strawberries, grapes, eggplant, carrots, green beans, kale, lettuce, tomatoes, lettuce, bell peppers

Low Fodmap Staples For Your Fridge:

Soft cheeses such as brie/camembert cheese, feta cheese, hard cheeses, lactose-free milk, mayonnaise, eggs, firm tofu, cooked meats/poultry/seafood

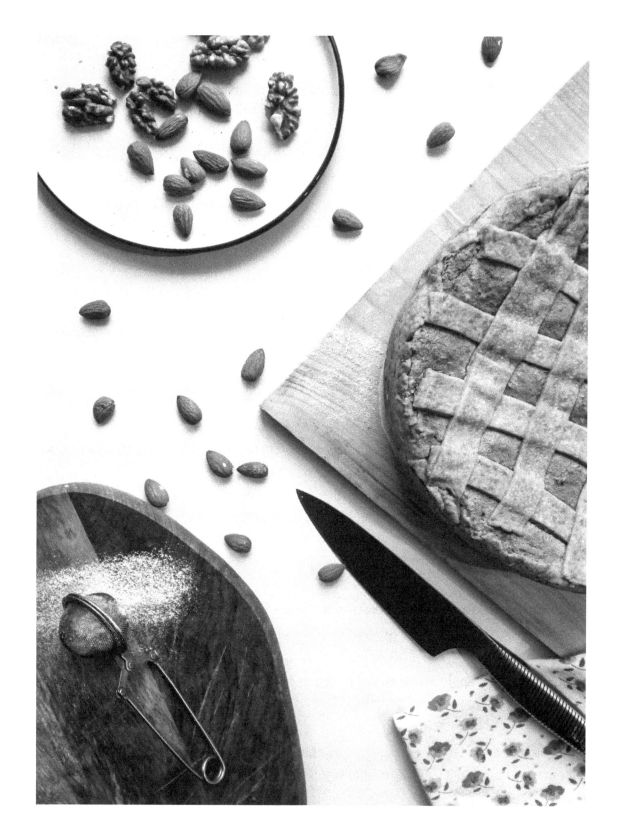

The Fodmap Diet Phases

The FODMAP diet has three phases, elimination, reintroduction, and maintenance. You'll start with the elimination phase.

Elimination Phase

It's recommended to follow this phase of the FODMAP diet for 2-6 weeks. For the elimination phase, follow my 4-week plan, or you can select recipes of your choosing from those in the book. All the recipes in my book are low in FODMAPs, so it doesn't matter which recipes you choose.

If your symptoms have disappeared after two weeks, then you can start on the next phase of the diet. Or if you need longer and you're using my 4-week plan, then you can rinse and repeat to continue the diet for up to 6 weeks.

As previously mentioned, if after six weeks, you see no improvement in your symptoms, then it's time to visit your physician.

As you know, IBS can also be triggered by stress. Unfortunately, IBS also CAUSES stress, so it can be a cyclical illness whereby having the disease causes you so much stress that it also gives you the illness. So, it can still be that a low FODMAP diet can help you in the future, but it may be that for now, you need to tackle your stress levels.

Reintroduction Phase

Once you have had time to get better, then you're ready to reintroduce foods one at a time. Now your symptoms have eased or disappeared; you can quickly identify which foods are triggering your IBS or other gut-related condition. You'll also follow a low FODMAP diet during the reintroduction phase too. So once again, if you're using my 4-week plan, then continue the diet for as many weeks as you like.

Just continue to reintroduce foods one at a time, over three days, allowing you to identify "culprit" foods that are making your gut poorly.

It's essential to make notes, or you can use a FODMAP app to help you do this. Make notes of the FODMAP group and the specific food each time. Once you have identified foods that trigger your symptoms, continue to eliminate them. If you tolerate them well, you can continue to enjoy them as part of a healthy diet.

It's as simple as that.

You keep adding different foods, and this way, you'll soon have built up more and more foods that you can tolerate. You may as well reintroduce your favorite foods first, one at a time rather than random foods.

The maintenance phase is just a case of continuing from the reintroduction phase. By now, you'll know if you can tolerate lactose in milk, for example, then you can adapt the recipes given in the book to include butter, cream, and milk, for example. Or go back to your old recipes that contain those ingredients now you know you can tolerate that ingredient without any symptoms.

It's important to note that just because you can't tolerate a certain food right now, you may be able to tolerate it later down the line. So it's worth reintroducing certain foods that you previously found triggered your symptoms at a later date.

There are so many alternatives to high FODMAP foods and so many delicious recipes to enjoy that you really can beat your symptoms and enjoy great food.

IBS is a real pain in the gut, if you'll pardon the pun and living with it can make life a misery. But with these delicious recipes and easy-to-follow diet plan, you could soon be IBS-free just like millions of IBS sufferers who have finally identified their food intolerances with the low FODMAP diet.

The one thing to mention is that no IBS sufferer is the same. The list of food intolerances a person has tends to be unique to each person. But once you have identified them and found tasty alternatives, you'll be amazed at how happy and healthy you finally feel now your symptoms are under control.

Best of luck!

Your 4-Week Low Fodmap Diet Plan

	Mon	Tues	Wed	Thurs	Fri	Sat	Sun
Breakfast	Carrot, Oat & Raisin Porridge	Cranberry & Almond Muesli	Gluten-Free Gingersnap Granola	Acai Bowl with Fruits	Banana & Oat Smoothie	Quinoa Porridge with Yogurt and Banana	Tomato & Mozzarella Breakfast Tortillas
Lunch	Cheesy Broccoli & Zucchini Fritters	Vegetable Fried Rice	Mustard Salmon Jar Salad	Spaghetti all' Amatriciana	Thai Pumpkin Noodle Soup	BLT Blue Cheese Omelet	Lemon-Butter Tilapia
Dinner	Campfire Salmon	Beef & Leek Stew	Chicken Wings	Grilled Swordfish	Beef Burgers with BBQ Sauce	Pork Loin with Maple Mustard Sauce	Beef Stroganoff
Dessert	Fruit Salad	Strawberry Frozen Yogurt	Milk Chocolate Chunk Cookies	Peanut Energy Bar	Rhubarb & Custard Cups	Blueberry Crumble Slice	Lemon Cake

	Mon	Tues	Wed	Thurs	Fri	Sat	Sun
Breakfast	Acai Bowl with Fruits	Carrot, Oat & Raisin Porridge	Quinoa Porridge with Yogurt and Banana	Cranberry & Almond Muesli	Gluten-Free Gingersnap Granola	Tomato & Mozzarella Breakfast Tortillas	Banana & Oat Smoothie
Lunch	Pumpkin & Carrot Risotto	Bacon & Egg Salad	Vegetable & Chickpea Soup	Simple Lamb Stew	Slow Cooker Chicken Soup	Salmon Fried Rice	Gorgonzola Penne
Dinner	Slow Cooker Herby Turkey	Spaghetti Bolognese	Spicy Chicken Drumsticks	Snapper with Chips	Chicken Saagwala	Dover Sole with Thyme	Espresso Ribeye
Dessert	Berry & Yogurt Mini Pavlovas	Chocolate & Cranberry Muesli Bar	Banana Bread	Strawberry Frozen Yogurt	Peanut Butter Cookies	Almond Muffins with Blueberry	Cream Cheese Brownies

	Mon	Tues	Wed	Thurs	Fri	Sat	Sun
Breakfast	Banana & Oat Smoothie	Quinoa Porridge with Yogurt and Banana	Carrot, Oat & Raisin Porridge	Acai Bowl with Fruits	Cranberry & Almond Muesli	Gluten-Free Gingersnap Granola	Tomato & Mozzarella Breakfast Tortillas
Lunch	Mustard Salmon Jar Salad	Thai Pumpkin Noodle Soup	Vegetable Fried Rice	Cheesy Broccoli & Zucchini Fritters	Beef & Leek Stew	Tuna & Sun-Dried Tomato Rigatoni	Slow Cooker Chicken Soup

Dinner	Snapper with Chips	Slow Cooker Herby Turkey	Sweet Potato & Lamb Fritters with Salad	Beef Stroganoff	Grilled Swordfish	Espresso Ribeye	Bacon-Wrapped Pork Loin
Dessert	Rhubarb & Custard Cups	Lemon Cake	Peanut Energy Bars	Dark Chocolate & Raspberry Pudding	Cantaloupe Lime Popsicles	Milk Chocolate Chunk Cookies	Almond Muffins with Blueberry

	Mon	Tues	Wed	Thurs	Fri	Sat	Sun
Breakfast	Banana & Oat Smoothie	Acai Bowl with Fruits	Tomato & Mozzarella Breakfast Tortillas	Carrot, Oat & Raisin Porridge	Quinoa Porridge with Yogurt and Banana	Cranberry & Almond Muesli	Gluten-Free Gingersnap Granola
Lunch	Salmon Fried Rice	Vegetable & Chickpea Soup	Simple Lamb Stew	Carrot & Fennel Soup	Sweet Red Pepper Soup	Spaghetti all' Amatriciana	Pasta Salad with Chickpeas & Feta
Dinner	Beef Burgers with BBQ Sauce	Campfire Salmon	Chicken Wings	Dover Sole with Thyme	Spaghetti Bolognese	Peanut Chicken Satay	Pork Loin with Maple Mustard Sauce
Dessert	Coconut Popsicles	Blueberry Crumble Slice	Cream Cheese Brownies	Peanut Butter Cookies	Lemon Blueberry Traybake	Strawberry Frozen Yogurt	Berry & Yogurt Mini Pavlovas

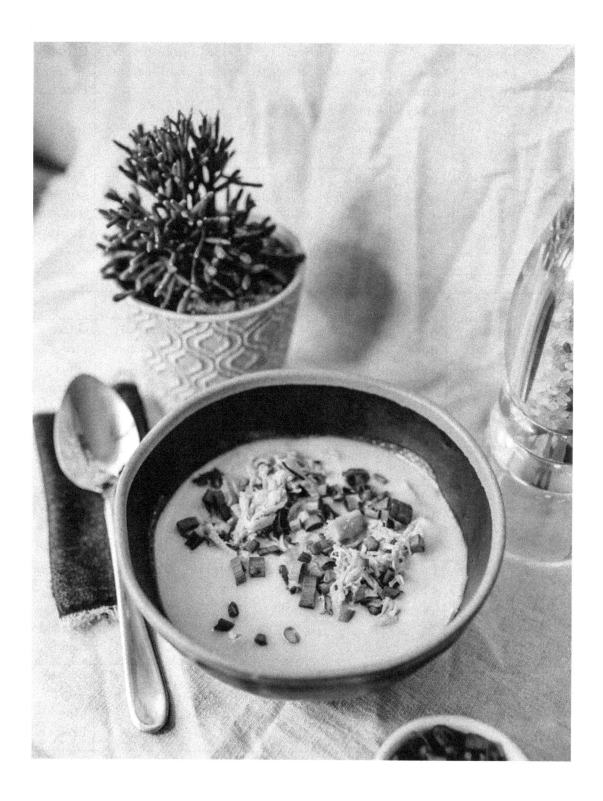

Chapter 3 Your Complete FODMAP Food Bible

As I've pointed out, IBS is a bit of a mystery. It's a case of working out what you are eating that is triggering your symptoms. And it stands to reason that it might be some of your favorite foods that are causing you problems. While that sounds like bad news, the good news is that there are so many alternatives.

Here's a complete list of foods you can and can't eat. There sometimes doesn't appear to be a great deal of logic as to why pecans are okay, and pistachios aren't, for example. So if you want to adapt your recipes or have a snack, then this complete list is here to refer to time and time again.

Food To Eat And Avoid

High Fodmap Fruits To Avoid:

- Apples
- Apricots
- Avocado
- Bananas, ripe
- Blackberries
- Blackcurrants
- Boysenberry
- Cherries
- Grapefruit
- Lychee
- Mango
- Nectarines, Peaches
- Pears
- Pineapple, dried
- Plums
- Pomegranate
- Raisins, Sultanas, Currants, Dates, Figs & Prunes
- Watermelon

LOW FODMAP Fruits To Eat:

- Bananas, unripe
- Berries, including Bilberries, Blueberries, Raspberries, Strawberries, Cranberries
- Citrus fruits including lemons, limes, oranges, & mandarin
- Dragon fruit
- Grapes
- Guava, ripe
- Honeydew, Cantaloupe, and Galia melons
- Kiwifruit
- Passion fruit
- Pawpaw
- Papaya
- Pineapple
- Plantain
- Rhubarb

Vegetables & Legumes To Avoid:

- Garlic including garlic salt, garlic powder
- Onions, including onion powder and small pickled onions
- Artichoke
- Asparagus
- Beans including baked, broad, butter, haricot, kidney, soy, lima and mung
- Beetroot, fresh
- Black-eyed peas
- Cauliflower
- Celery
- Leek bulb
- Mange Tout
- Mushrooms
- Peas
- Pickled vegetables
- Savoy Cabbage
- Split peas
- Scallions, white part
- Shallots

LOW FODMAP Vegetables Good To Eat:

- Alfalfa
- Bamboo shoots
- Bean sprouts
- Bell pepper
- Beetroot
- Black beans
- Bok choy
- Broccoli
- Butternut squash
- Cabbage
- Carrots
- Celeriac
- Celery
- Chicory leaves
- Chickpeas
- Chili
- Chives
- Collard greens
- Courgette
- Cucumber
- Eggplant
- Fennel
- Green beans
- Ginger
- Kale
- Karela
- Leek leaves
- Lettuce:
- Marrow
- Okra
- Olives
- Parsnip
- Pickled gherkins
- Potato
- Pumpkin
- Radish
- Scallions, green part
- Seaweed
- Spaghetti squash
- Spinach, baby
- Squash
- Swede
- Swiss chard
- Sweet potato
- Tomato
- Turnip
- Water chestnuts
- Yam
- Zucchini

HIGH FODMAP Meats, Poultry And Meat Substitutes To Avoid:

- Chorizo
- Sausages

LOW FODMAP Meats, Poultry, and Meat SubstituteS TO EAT:

- Beef
- Chicken
- Kangaroo
- Lamb
- Pork
- Prosciutto
- Quorn, mince
- Turkey
- Cold cuts/deli meat / cold meats such as ham and turkey breast
- Processed meat – check ingredients

LOW FODMAP Fish and Seafood To Eat:

- Canned tuna
- Whitefish such as Cod, Haddock & Snapper
- Oily fish such as Salmon, Mackerel
- River fish such as Trout
- Seafood such as Crab, Lobster, Mussels, Oysters & Shrimp

HIGH FODMAP Dairy Foods To Avoid:

- Buttermilk
- Cheeses including cream, Cheese, Halloumi, cheese, ricotta
- Cream
- Custard
- Gelato and Ice cream made with cow's milk
- Cow's milk, Goat's milk, Evaporated milk, Sheep's milk
- Sour cream
- Yogurt

- Butter
- Some cheeses including Brie, Camembert, Cheddar, Cottage, Feta, Goat's, Monterey Jack, Mozzarella, Parmesan, Swiss
- Dairy-free chocolate pudding
- Eggs
- Margarine
- Almond milk, Hemp milk, Lactose-free milk, Macadamia milk, & Rice milk
- Sorbet
- Soy protein
- Tempeh
- Tofu – drained and firm varieties
- Whipped cream
- Coconut yogurt, Lactose-free yogurt, Goats yogurt

- Wheat containing products such as biscuits, wheat-based bread, breadcrumbs, Cakes, Muffins, Pastries, Croissants
- Egg noodles
- Pasta and gnocchi
- Wheat bran
- Wheat-based breakfast cereals including muesli
- Wheat flour
- Wheat germ
- Almond meal
- Barley
- Bran cereals
- Cashews
- Couscous
- Pistachios
- Rye
- Semolina

- Wheat-free and Gluten-free bread including Cornbread, Oat bread, Rice bread, Spelt sourdough bread & Potato flour bread
- Wheat-free or Gluten-free pasta
- Bulgur
- Buckwheat including flour, noodles
- Brazil nuts, chestnuts, hazelnuts, macadamia, peanuts, pecans, pine nuts, almonds, walnuts
- Chips, plain / potato crisps, plain
- Crispbread
- Corn cakes
- Cornflakes, Gluten-free
- Coconut – milk, cream, flesh
- Corn, creamed and canned (up to 1/3 cup)
- Corn tortillas
- Crackers, plain
- Millet
- Oatmeal, Oats, & Oatcakes
- Polenta
- Popcorn
- Porridge and oat-based cereals
- Potato flour
- Pretzels
- Quinoa
- Rice, including Basmati rice, Brown rice, Rice noodles. White rice, Rice bran, Rice cakes. Rice crackers, Rice flakes, Rice flour & Rice Krispies
- Seeds including Chia, Hemp, Flax, Poppy, Pumpkin, Sesame & Sunflower
- Maize, potato, and tapioca starch
- Tortilla chips/corn chips

- Beer
- Coconut water
- Cordial
- Fruit and herbal teas with apple added
- Fruit juices in large quantities
- Fruit juices made of apple, pear, mango, orange
- Malted chocolate-flavored drink
- Meal replacement drinks containing milk-based products
- Sodas containing High Fructose Corn Syrup
- Soy milk
- Sports drinks
- Tea, including Chai, Dandelion, Fennel. Chamomile, Herbal, Oolong
- Wine
- Whey protein, unless lactose-free

HIGH FODMAP Condiments, Dips, Sweets, Sweeteners and Spreads To Avoid:

- Agave, honey, Molasses, Honey, Sweeteners including Maltitol, Sorbitol, Xylitol,
- Jam
- Pesto sauce
- Relish/vegetable pickle
- Stock cubes
- Sugar-free sweets containing polyols – usually ending in -ol or isomalt
- Tahini paste
- Tzatziki dip

LOW FODMAP Condiments, Dips, Sweets, Sweeteners and Spreads to Eat:

- Almond butter
- Barbecue sauce
- Capers
- Chocolate in small quantities
- Dijon mustard
- Fish sauce
- Ketchup
- Marmalade
- Mayonnaise
- Miso paste
- Mustard
- Oyster sauce
- Peanut butter
- Soy sauce
- Sweet and sour sauce
- Sugar, Stevia, Saccharine, Rice malt syrup, Maple syrup, Golden syrup, Erythritol, Aspartame, Acesulfame K
- Tamarind paste
- Tomato sauce
- Vinegar including Apple cider, Balsamic & Rice wine vinegar
- Wasabi
- Worcestershire sauce

What About Garlic And Onions?

You may have noticed that garlic and onions are on the avoid list. Many people love garlic and onions are the base to nearly every savory dish you can think of. However, they are irritant and are off-limits, at least for now, during the low FODMAP few weeks. That doesn't mean they'll be off-limits forever. That being said, if you have symptoms all the time, then it's entirely feasible you are intolerant to these classic flavor enhancers.

If you love garlic in your food as well as onion, then you can try introducing them straightaway at the reintroduction phase. That way, you'll be able to find out if you can tolerate them or not.

However, there are plenty of other ways to add garlic and onion flavors to popular foods. You can use garlic-infused oil to add that delicious garlicky flavor to your favorite foods. You can even make garlic bread using garlic-flavored oil (see page XX).

For other dishes, the "onion flavor" is added by using leek leaves or the green parts of scallions to dishes. These are still part of the "onion family" but are low in FODMAPs.

Low Fodmap Recipes Store Cupboard

- Oil including vegetable, sesame, olive, and garlic-infused olive oil
- Herbs
- Spices
- Eggs
- Seeds, including flax, hemp, chia, and sesame
- Flours including gluten-free all-purpose flour,
- LOW FODMAP sugar and sweetener including granulated and liquid Stevia powder/maple syrup/rice malt syrup, white, brown and confectioner's sugar
- Peanut butter
- Tinned tomatoes
- Sun-dried tomatoes
- Low FODMAP oyster sauce
- Low FODMAP hot sauce
- Mayonnaise
- Worcestershire sauce
- BBQ sauce
- Mustard, Dijon, and mustard powder
- Lemon juice
- Canned beetroot
- Tomato paste
- Gluten-free pasta
- Gluten-free bread
- Low FODMAP stock
- Rice
- Thai Fish sauce
- Ginger
- Quinoa flakes
- Oats
- Balsamic vinegar
- Salt and pepper

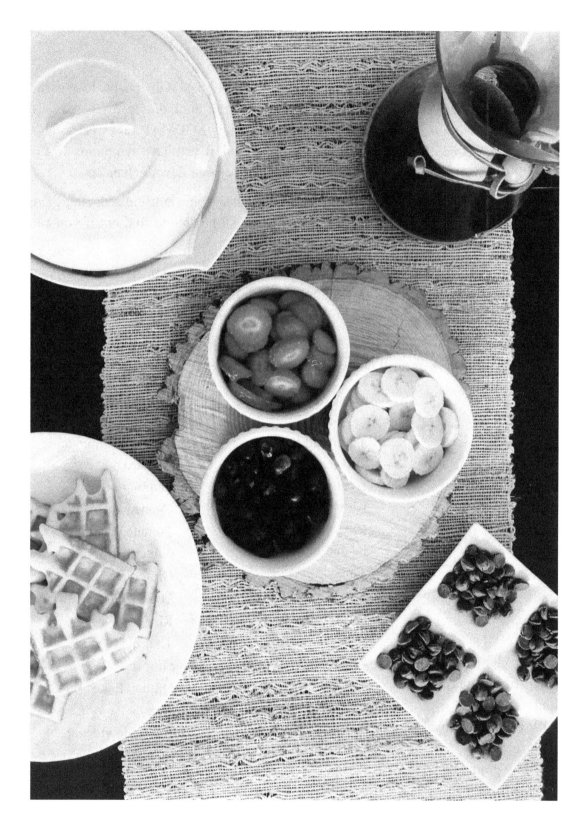

Carrot, Oat & Raisin Porridge

Prep time: 5 minutes, cook time: 12 minutes; Serves 4

5 Ingredients

- 1 cup oats
- 2 medium carrots, grated
- ¼ cup raisins
- ¼ cup walnuts
- ½ cup milk

What you'll need from the store cupboard:

- 1 tsp cinnamon
- 1 tbsp flax seeds
- 4 tbsp hemp seeds

Instructions:

1. Take a medium pot and add oats and water, stir it on medium heat.

2. When the mixture comes to the boil, then add carrots to it while stirring.

3. After approximately 12 minutes of cooking, turn the heat off and add other dried fruits into it.

4. Serve with maple syrup

Nutrition Facts Per Serving

Calories 288, Total Fat 10g, Saturated Fat 2g, Total Carbs 30g, Net Carbs 24g, Protein 10g, Sugar 12g, Fiber 6g, Sodium 55mg.

Cranberry & Almond Muesli

5 Ingredients

- 20 whole almonds
- 1 tbsp dried cranberries
- ½ cup coconut milk

What you'll need from the store cupboard:

- 1 cup of boiled oats
- 2 tbsp pumpkin seeds
- ½ cup water

- 2 tsp cinnamon
- 1 tsp of vanilla extract
- Pinch of low sodium salt

Instructions:

1. Place oats and almonds in a food processor and pulse until fine.

2. Place all ingredients in a large bowl and stir well.

3. Place in refrigerator and leave to swell overnight.

4. In the morning you can loosen the porridge with extra milk if desired.

Nutrition Facts Per Serving

Calories 366, Total Fat 16g, Saturated Fat 3g, Total Carbs 38g, Net Carbs 33g, Protein 12g, Sugar 5g, Fiber 5g, Sodium 26mg

Acai Bowl with Fruits

5 Ingredients

- 2 tbsp acai powder
- ½ cup raspberries
- 1 cup of strawberries
- 1 small bunch of spinach
- ½ cup of coconut milk

What you' ll need from the store cupboard:

- 1 tsp hemp seeds
- 1 tsp maple syrup
- 1 tsp vanilla extract
- 1 tsp natural peanut butter
- Pinch of low sodium salt

Instructions:

1. Place all ingredients into a blender and blitz.

2. Season to taste with salt if desired.

3. Pour it into a bowl and top with fruit toppings such as kiwi, pineapple and more fresh berries.

4. Serve immediately.

Nutrition Facts Per Serving

Calories 507, Total Fat 23g, Saturated Fat 3g, Total Carbs 42g, Net Carbs 27g, Protein 12g, Sugar 24g, Fiber 16g, Sodium 200mg

Tomato & Mozzarella Breakfast Tortillas

Prep time: 20 minutes, cook time: 5 minutes; Serves 4

5 Ingredients

- 4 corn tortillas
- 4 eggs, hard-boiled and sliced
- 1 cup mozzarella
- ½ cup natural yogurt

What you' ll need from the store cupboard:

- 1 tsp ginger
- 1 tsp garlic-infused oil
- 1 tsp olive oil
- Pinch of low sodium salt

Instructions:

1. Heat the oil in a large pan and quickly fry the tortillas.

2. Mix yogurt, cheese, diced tomatoes and eggs, and pile onto the tortillas.

3. Season to taste and wrap up burrito-style for breakfast on the go.

Nutrition Facts Per Serving

Calories 259, Total Fat 13g, Saturated Fat 6g, Total Carbs 14g, Net Carbs 9g, Protein 18g, Sugar 6g, Fiber 5g, Sodium 178mg

Quinoa Porridge with Yogurt and Banana

Prep time: 15 minutes, cook time: 10 minutes; Serves 1

5 Ingredients

- ⅓ ripe banana
- 3 tbsp lactose-free yogurt
- 1 cup lactose-free milk

What you' ll need from the store cupboard:

- ⅓ cup quinoa flakes
- Sprinkle of cinnamon
- 1 tsp vanilla extract
- 1 tsp maple syrup
- ½ cup water
- Pinch of salt

Instructions:

1. Boil water and milk in a pan and then add the quinoa flakes.

2. Boil for 5 minutes and then reduce to a simmer for 2 minutes.

3. Stir in yogurt, banana, maple syrup, and salt.

3. Sprinkle with cinnamon and serve immediately.

Nutrition Facts Per Serving

Calories 468, Total Fat 9g, Saturated Fat 4g, Total Carbs 76g, Net Carbs 70g, Protein 19g, Sugar: 38g, Fiber: 7g, Sodium 150 mg.

Gluten-Free Gingersnap Granola

5 Ingredients

- 3 cups old-fashioned rolled oats
- 1 tbsp dried ground ginger
- 3 tbsp finely grated fresh peeled ginger
- ½ cup sliced almonds

What you ' ll need from the store cupboard:

- ¼ tsp salt
- ¼ tsp cinnamon
- ⅓ cup maple syrup
- ⅓ cup light brown sugar
- ⅔ cup vegetable oil
- 1 cup quinoa flakes

Instructions:

1. Preheat oven to 325°F.

2. Combine all ingredients in a large bowl and mix well.

3. Spread the granola out onto a baking sheet.

4. Bake for around 15 minutes, stirring halfway through to ensure even cooking.

5. Cool before storing in an airtight container. Serve with yogurt or milk.

Nutrition Facts Per Serving

Calories 227, Total Fat 9g, Saturated Fat 1g, Total Carbs 32g, Net Carbs 28g, Protein 5g, Sugar: 5g, Fiber: 4g, Sodium 27mg.

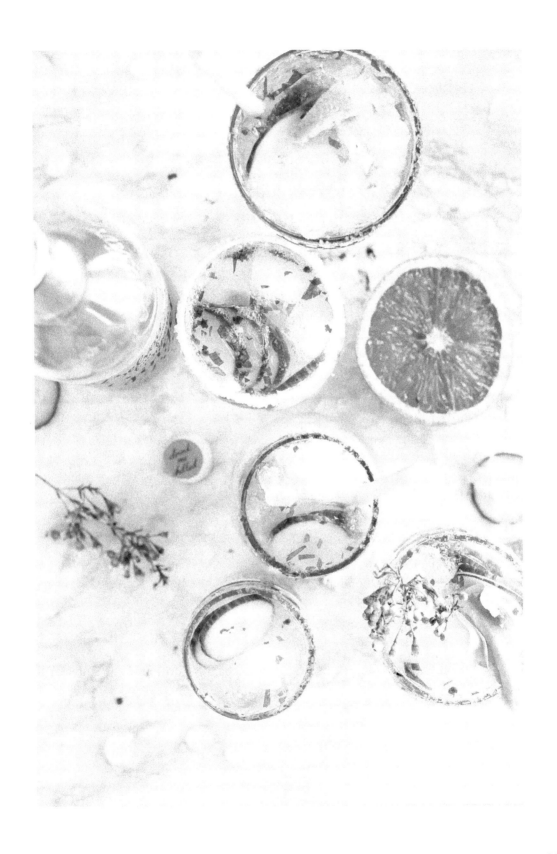

Banana & Oat Smoothie

Prep time: 5 minutes, cook time: 12 minutes; Serves 1

5 Ingredients

- 1 banana
- ½ cup unsweetened almond milk
- ¼ cup low-fat Greek yogurt
- ½ cup coconut milk

What you' ll need from the store cupboard:

- ¼ cup rolled oats
- ½ tsp vanilla essence
- 1 pinch of cinnamon
- 1 pinch of nutmeg
- ½ maple syrup
- ½ tsp liquid sweetener

Instructions:

1. Place all the ingredients in the blender and blitz until smooth.

2. Serve immediately.

Nutrition Facts Per Serving

Calories 239, Total Fat 4g, Total Carbs 36g, Net Carbs 30g, Protein 11g, Sugars 18g, Fiber 6g, Sodium 81mg

Blueberry, Banana & Chia Smoothie

5 Ingredients

- 2 tsp rice protein powder
- ¼ cup frozen banana
- ¼ cup vanilla soy ice cream (or lactose-free ice cream or lactose-free yogurt)
- ½ cup low FODMAP milk
- ½ cup blueberries

What you' ll need from the store cupboard:

- 1 tsp chia seeds
- 1 tsp lemon juice
- ½ tbsp maple syrup
- 6 ice cubes

Instructions:

1. Place all ingredients in a blender and blitz well.

2. Pour into a serving glass and serve immediately.

Nutrition Facts Per Serving

Calories 308, Total Fat 10 g, Saturated Fat 1.5g g, Total Carbs 50 g, Net Carbs 45g, Sugar 31 g, Fiber 5 g, Protein 6 g, Sodium 80mg.

Berries & Cream Smoothie

5 Ingredients

- 1 tsp lemon juice

- 1 cup strawberries, fresh or frozen, chopped

- ½ cup low FODMAP milk

- 1 cup blueberries, fresh or frozen

What you' ll need from the store cupboard:

- ¼ cup vanilla soy ice cream (or lactose-free ice cream or lactose-free yogurt)

- 2 tsp rice protein powder

- 1 tsp chia seeds

- ½ tbsp maple syrup

- 6 ice cubes

Instructions:

1. Place all ingredients in a blender.

2. If you are using fresh berries add ice cubes but omit if using frozen ones.

3. Blitz until well blended.

4. Pour into a serving glass and drink immediately.

Nutrition Facts Per Serving

Calories 308, Total Fat 10 g, Saturated Fat 1g g, Total Carbs 49 g, Net Carbs 43g, Sugar 31 g, Fiber 6 g, Protein 5 g, Sodium 80mg.

Virgin Piña Colada

5 Ingredients

- 1 cup fresh pineapple, cut into rough chunks
- ½ cup coconut milk
- 1 cup frozen banana

What you'll need from the store cupboard:

- 1½ cup water
- ⅓ cup sugar
- 1 tsp vanilla extract

Instructions:

1. Make sugar water by heating the water and sugar in a saucepan until sugar dissolves. Set aside and chill.

2. When sugar water is chilled, place all the ingredients in a blender and blitz until well blended.

3. Pour into serving glasses and serve immediately.

Nutrition Facts Per Serving

Calories 207, Total Fat 7g, Saturated Fat 6g, Total Carbs 38g, Net Carbs 37g, Sugar 29g, Fiber 1g, Protein 1g, Sodium 0mg.

Strawberry Mimosa Fizz

5 Ingredients

- 1 bottle of sparkling wine or champagne
- 1 cup fresh strawberries, chopped

What you' ll need from the store cupboard:

- ½ cup sugar
- ¾ cup water

Instructions:

1. Make sugar water by heating the water and sugar in a saucepan until sugar dissolves. Set aside and chill.

2. Blitz the strawberries and sugar syrup in a blender.

3. Pour 2 tablespoons of strawberry syrup into champagne flutes and top with your chosen fizz.

4. Serve immediately.

Nutrition Facts Per Serving

Calories 133, Total Fat 0 g, Saturated Fat 0g, Total Carbs 18g, Net Carbs 18g, Sugar 14g, Fiber 0g, Protein 0g, Sodium 0mg.

Good Old-fashioned Mint Lemonade Cooler

5 Ingredients

- 2 cup fresh lemon juice

- 1 handful fresh mint, chopped

What you' ll need from the store cupboard:

- 1½ cup sugar

- 6½ cup water

Instructions:

1. Make sugar water by heating the 1½ cups of water and sugar in a saucepan until sugar dissolves. Set aside and chill.

2. Place the lemon juice and remaining water into a large jug.

3. Add the sugar syrup to taste.

4. Stir in the mint.

5. The lemonade will keep in a sealed jug for up to 1 week.

Nutrition Facts Per Serving

Calories 84, Total Fat 0g, Saturated Fat 0g, Total Carbs 22g, Net Carbs 22g, Sugar 20g, Fiber 0g, Protein 0g, Sodium 0mg.

Hot Lemon, Ginger & Maple Drink

5 Ingredients

- 1 unwaxed lemon, sliced

- 1 tbsp fresh ginger, thinly sliced

What you' ll need from the store cupboard:

- ½ cup maple syrup

Instructions:

1. Place all the ingredients in layers in a jar.

2. Refrigerate overnight.

3. Add a spoonful of lemon ginger syrup to hot water in a mug for a soothing drink, when desired.

4. The syrup will keep for several weeks in the refrigerator.

Nutrition Facts Per Serving

Calories 30, Total Fat 0g, Saturated Fat 0g, Total Carbs 78g, Net Carbs 8g, Sugar 6g, Fiber 0g, Protein 0g, Sodium 0mg.

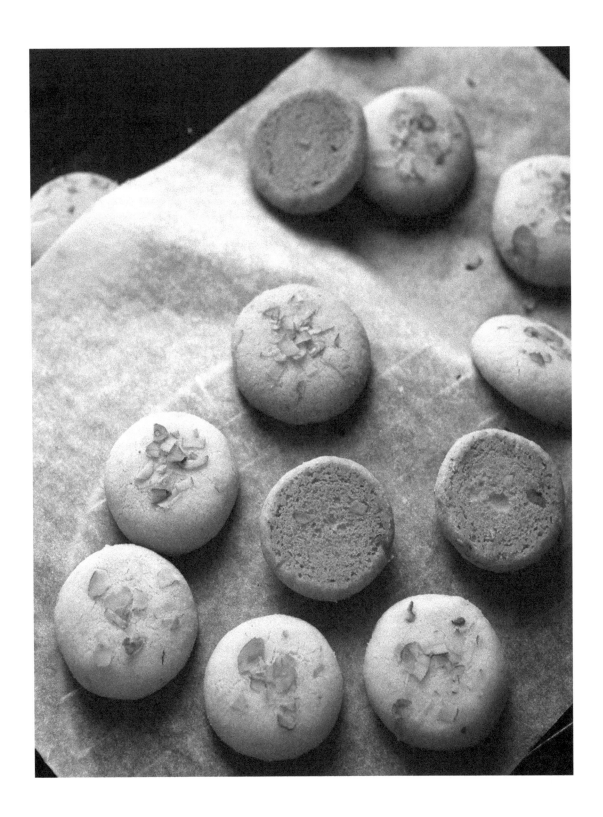

Chocolate & Espresso Power Balls

Prep time: 10 minutes, cook time: 0 minutes: Serves 12

5 Ingredients

- ¼ cup chocolate-covered espresso beans, crushed

- 2 tsp instant powdered espresso

- 4 tsp Dutch-processed cocoa

- ⅓ cup rice syrup

What you' ll need from the store cupboard:

- ⅛ teaspoon vanilla extract

- 1 cup old-fashioned oats

- ½ cup creamy peanut butter

Instructions:

1. Place all the ingredients except the crushed chocolate-covered espresso beans into a large bowl and mix well until evenly combined.

2. Fold in the espresso beans and chill in the refrigerator for 30 minutes.

3. Roll the mixture into bite-sized balls about 1-inch in diameter. The mixture should make 12 balls.

4. Store in the refrigerator for a week or freeze for up to a month.

Nutrition Facts Per Serving

Calories 174, Total Fat 8g, Saturated Fat 1g, Total Carbs 22g, Net Carbs 19g, Sugar 6g, Fiber 3g, Protein 6g, Sodium 0mg.

White Chocolate & Cranberry Energy Balls

5 Ingredients

- ⅓ cup maple syrup or rice syrup
- ½ cup dried cranberries, coarsely chopped
- ⅔ cup white chocolate chips

What you' ll need from the store cupboard:

- ½ cup natural peanut butter
- 1 cup old-fashioned oats
- ⅛ tsp vanilla extract

Instructions:

1. Place all the ingredients into a large bowl and mix well until evenly combined.

2. Chill in the refrigerator for 30 minutes.

3. Roll the mixture into bite-sized balls about 1-inch in diameter. The mixture should make 12 balls.

4. Store in the refrigerator for a week or freeze for up to a month.

Nutrition Facts Per Serving

Calories 243, Total Fat 9g, Saturated Fat 1g, Total Carbs 37g, Net Carbs 34g, Sugar 21g, Fiber 3g, Protein 6g, Sodium 0mg.

BLT Blue Cheese Omelet

Prep time: 5 minutes, cook time: 5 minutes; Serves 2

5 Ingredients

- 4 large eggs, beaten
- 8 cherry or grape tomatoes, halved
- 4 rashers of crisp bacon, crumbled or chopped into bite-sized pieces
- 2oz blue cheese
- Handful of baby lettuce

What you' ll need from the store cupboard:

- 1 tbsp water
- 1 tbsp oil
- Salt and freshly ground black pepper

Instructions:

1. Whisk all the ingredients in a bowl except for the oil.

2. Heat the oil until hot in a large non-stick skillet and pour in the mixture.

3. Cook the omelet until it is beginning to set. As it sets, use a heat-proof spatula to fold the edges in and away from the side of the skillet.

4. Once the omelet is almost dry fold it in half and slide onto a serving plate.

Nutrition Facts Per Serving

Calories 301, Total Fat 23g, Saturated Fat 0g, Total Carbs 2g, Net Carbs 2g, Sugar 1g, Fiber 0g, Protein 18g, Sodium 120mg.

Garlic Infused Croutons

5 Ingredients

- 8 slices gluten-free bread, cut into ½ to 1-inch cubes
- 3 tbsp dairy-free spread

What you' ll need from the store cupboard:

- 4 tsp garlic-infused oil
- ½ tsp dried oregano
- Pinch of salt

Instructions:

1. Preheat the oven to 340ºF.

2. Melt the dairy-free spread and garlic-infused oil in a bowl in the microwave for 10-20 seconds on HIGH.

4. Add croutons to the bowl and toss them through to evenly coat.

5. Spread the croutons in a single layer on a baking tray and sprinkle over the oregano and salt.

6. Bake for 10 to 15 minutes, turning once to prevent over-browning.

7. Store in an airtight container and serve as a snack or on top of soups and salads.

Nutrition Facts Per Serving

Calories 285, Total Fat 15g, Saturated Fat 2g, Total Carbs 32g, Net Carbs 31g, Sugar 3g, Fiber 1g, Protein 6.5g, Sodium 200mg.

Curly Fries

Prep time: 20 minutes, cook time: 25 minutes; Serves 4

5 Ingredients

- 1½lb potatoes, peeled

What you' ll need from the store cupboard:

- 2 tbsp vegetable oil
- ½ tsp paprika
- Dried chili flakes
- Salt and freshly ground black pepper

Instructions:

1. Preheat the oven to 400ºF.

2. Put the potatoes through a spiralizer.

3. Spread the potato spirals out onto two baking trays.

4. Drizzle with oil and sprinkle with salt, pepper, paprika, and chili flakes.

5. Toss the fries to ensure they are evenly coated then bake for 20-25 minutes.

6. Shake the fries halfway through cooking.

7. Serve hot with your favorite entrees or as a snack with ketchup.

Nutrition Facts Per Serving

Calories 185, Total Fat 3g, Saturated Fat 0g, Total Carbs 37g, Net Carbs 32g, Sugar 2g, Fiber 5g, Protein 4g, Sodium 40mg.

Dutch Pancake

5 Ingredients

- 2 large eggs, beaten
- ½ cup lactose-free whole milk
- Blueberries, raspberries or strawberries
- 1 tsp lemon juice

What you' ll need from the store cupboard:

- 2 tsp water
- 1 tsp confectioners' sugar
- Pinch Kosher salt
- ½ cup gluten-free flour

Instructions:

1. Preheat oven to 450°F.

2. Whisk milk, flour, and salt into the beaten eggs.

3. Melt butter in a 10 to 12-inch ovenproof skillet. When hot pour in the batter.

4. Place the skillet in the oven and reduce the heat to 425°F.

5. Bake for 12-15 minutes until the pancake is puffed and golden.

6. Sprinkle with lemon juice and sugar and serve immediately.

Nutrition Facts Per Serving

Calories 172, Total Fat 9g, Saturated Fat 0g, Total Carbs 17g, Net Carbs 16g, Sugar 2g, Fiber 1g, Protein 5g, Sodium 30mg.

Crunchy Low FODMAP Garlic Bread

5 Ingredients

- 6 slices bread, sliced into triangles
- 4 tbsp dairy-free spread

What you' ll need from the store cupboard:

- Salt
- 1 tsp dried oregano
- 3 tbsp garlic-infused oil

Instructions:

1. Melt the dairy-free spread (or you can use butter) in the microwave on HIGH for around 20 seconds.

2. Place the bread on a baking tray and brush with melted spread using a pastry brush.

3. Sprinkle with salt and oregano.

4. Place under the grill until golden. Then turn the bread and brush with remaining garlic spread.

5. Grill again for 2 more minutes and serve immediately as a snack or with a gluten-free pasta meal such as Spaghetti Bolognese.

Nutrition Facts Per Serving

Calories 212, Total Fat 15g, Saturated Fat 2g, Total Carbs 16g, Net Carbs 15g, Sugar 1g, Fiber 1g, Protein 3g, Sodium 120mg.

Quick & Easy Gumdrops

5 Ingredients

- 3 envelopes unflavored gelatin
- Red food coloring

What you'll need from the store cupboard:

- 1¼ cup water
- 1½ cup sugar plus extra to coat
- ½ tsp fruit-flavored extract

Instructions:

1. Allow the gelatin to dissolve in half a cup of water for 5 minutes.

2. Place the remaining water and sugar in a saucepan and bring to the boil, stirring all the time.

3. Add gelatin mixture and reduce heat to a simmer. Cook for 5 minutes, stirring frequently.

4. Remove from heat and stir in the food coloring and flavoring.

5. Pour the mixture into a greased 8-in square pan, cover and refrigerate.

6. After 3 hours, turn the slab out onto a sugared board. Slice into 64 cubes and coat in sugar.

7. Store in an airtight container between parchment paper to prevent the gumdrops from sticking together.

Nutrition Facts Per Serving

Calories 19, Total Fat 0g, Saturated Fat 0g, Total Carbs 0g, Net Carbs 0g, Sugar 5g, Fiber 0g, Protein 0g, Sodium 1mg.

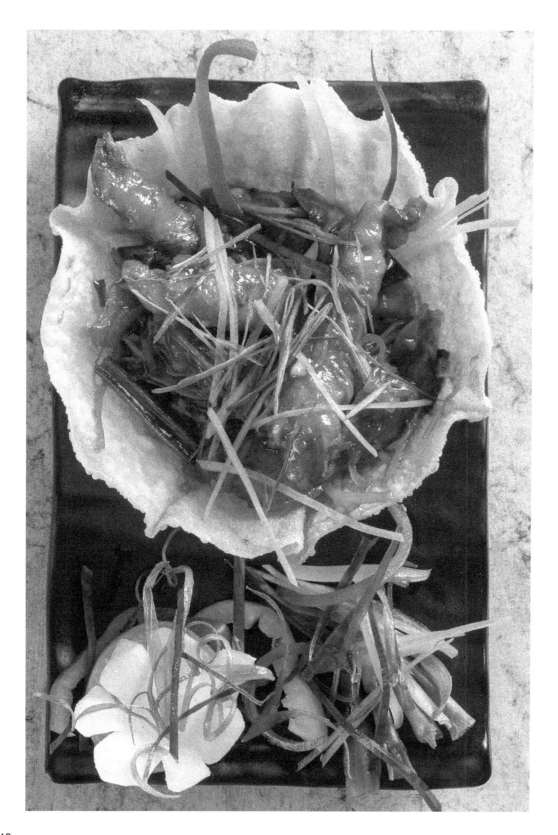

Chapter 7 Fish and Seafood Recipe

Dover Sole with Thyme & Parsley Butter

Prep time: 10 minutes, cook time: 35 minutes: Serves 4

5 Ingredients

- 4 Dover sole, cleaned and head removed

- 1 tbsp fresh thyme

- 1 tbsp fresh parsley

- ¼ cup salted butter

What you' ll need from the store cupboard:

- Salt and freshly ground black pepper

Instructions:

1. Preheat the oven to 375°F.

2. Season the fish with salt and freshly ground pepper.

3. Place the fish in a shallow dish and pour in water to around a ¼ inch depth.

4. Bake for 20 to 30 minutes, depending on the size of the fish.

4. While the fish is cooking make the herb butter by melting the butter in a small saucepan. Stir in the herbs.

5. Just before serving, make the herb butter: In a saucepan, gently melt the butter, then stir in freshly chopped herbs.

6. To serve, plate the fish and spoon over the herb butter.

Nutrition Facts Per Serving

Calories 169, Total Fat 5g, Saturated Fat 4g, Total Carbs 0g, Net Carbs 0g, Sugar 0g, Fiber 0g, Protein 31g, Sodium 6mg.

Grilled Swordfish with Tomato Olive Salsa

5 Ingredients

- 6 5oz swordfish steaks, ¾ inch to 1 inch thick
- 2 tbsp fresh flat-leaf parsley, chopped
- ½ cup pitted mixed Kalamata and green olives, chopped
- 1½ cup fresh plum tomatoes, cored, seeded and diced
- 2 tbsp fresh basil, chopped

What you' ll need from the store cupboard:

- 1 tbsp balsamic vinegar
- ½ tsp dried basil
- 8 tbsp garlic-infused oil
- 2 tbsp drained, brined small capers
- Salt and freshly ground black pepper

Instructions:

1. First make the salsa by combining the chopped tomatoes, 6 tablespoons of oil, olives, 1 tablespoon of basil, capers, and vinegar in a bowl. Season to taste with salt and pepper. Set aside for at least one hour to allow the flavors to amalgamate.

2. Make a marinade for the fish by blending the remaining oil and basil and lemon juice in a large bowl. Season with salt and pepper and allow the fish to marinate for 10 minutes.

3. Set the grill to high and grill the fish for approximately 3-4 minutes on each side.

4. Serve the fish with the salsa spooned over the top.

Nutrition Facts Per Serving

Calories 331, Total Fat 25g, Saturated Fat 0g, Total Carbs 2g, Net Carbs 2g, Sugar 1g, Fiber 0g, Protein 23g, Sodium 48mg.

Cod with Preserved Lemons & Basil

5 Ingredients

- 1lb cod loin, cut into 2 pieces
- ⅓ preserved lemon, chopped
- 3 tbsp fresh basil leaves, chopped
- 2 tbsp fresh parsley, chopped

What you' ll need from the store cupboard:

- 2 tbsp garlic-infused oil
- Salt and freshly ground black pepper

Instructions:

1. Preheat oven to 400°F.

2. Drizzle one tablespoon of the oil on the bottom of a large roasting pan.

3. Place fish in pan and season with salt and pepper. Scatter lemons and two tablespoons of the basil over the fish.

4. Drizzle with remaining oil and bake for approximately 10 minutes.

5. Serve immediately with remaining basil and parsley sprinkled over the top.

Nutrition Facts Per Serving

Calories 213, Total Fat 11g, Saturated Fat 0g, Total Carbs 1g, Net Carbs 1g, Sugar 0g, Fiber 0g, Protein 27g, Sodium 586mg.

Chilli Coconut Crusted Snapper with Chips

5 Ingredients

- 1lb Snapper or other mild white fish
- 1 tbsp mild green chilies, finely sliced
- 1 tbsp fresh lime zest

- 5 cup potato
- ½ cup Colby, cheddar cheese, or soy-free cheese, grated

What you' ll need from the store cupboard:

- 4 tbsp sesame oil
- ¼ cup dried shredded coconut
- 1 tbsp vegetable oil

- 1 lemon
- Salt & freshly ground black pepper

Instructions:

1. Leave the shredded coconut to soak in a bowl with water for 10 minutes.

2. Heat half of the sesame oil in a large skillet and fry the scallions.

3. Add chilies and coconut and fry for one minute. Remove from the pan and set aside.

4. Add the remaining sesame oil to the pan and cook the potatoes until golden in two batches. Season the chips with salt and pepper and keep warm.

5. In a separate skillet fry the fish for 2 minutes on each side in the vegetable oil.

5. Transfer the fish to a shallow baking dish and sprinkle over the cheese and top with coconut crust.

6. Grill the fish for 2 minutes until the crust is brown.

7. Make a basic salad of lettuce, tomatoes, and cucumbers to serve with your fish and chips.

Nutrition Facts Per Serving

Calories 486, Total Fat 21g, Saturated Fat 8g, Total Carbs 45g, Net Carbs 37g, Sugar 9g, Fiber 8g, Protein 34g, Sodium 80mg.

Sweet & Sticky Salmon Skewers

5 Ingredients

- 1lb fresh salmon fillets, skinned, deboned and cut into 1-inch cubes

- 1½ tsp crushed ginger

- 1 tbsp sesame seeds, toasted

- 1 large lime, zested and juiced

What you' ll need from the store cupboard:

- 2 tsp garlic-infused oil

- 1½ tbsp maple syrup

- 2 tbsp soy sauce

Instructions:

1. Place all the ingredients except the sesame seeds in a large bowl and leave to marinate for 10 minutes.

2. At the same time, place the wooden skewers in water to prevent them from burning.

3. Thread the salmon onto the skewers and place on an oiled tray.

4. Grill the skewers for 10 minutes turning frequently and basting with the marinade.

5. When cooked sprinkle the salmon skewers with toasted sesame seeds and serve.

Nutrition Facts Per Serving

Calories 197, Total Fat 8g, Saturated Fat 1g, Total Carbs 1g, Net Carbs 0g, Sugar 5g, Fiber 1g, Protein 22g, Sodium 240mg.

Lemon-Butter Tilapia with Almonds

5 Ingredients

- 4 4oz tilapia fillets
- 1¼ cup butter, cubed
- ¼ cup white wine or chicken broth
- 2 tbsp lemon juice
- ¼ cup sliced almonds

What you' ll need from the store cupboard:

- ½ tsp salt
- ¼ tsp pepper
- 1 tbsp olive oil

Instructions:

1. Season the fish with salt and pepper.

2. Heat the oil in a large skillet. Cook fish for 2-3 minutes on each side. Set aside and keep warm.

3. Place the butter, wine, and lemon juice to the same pan. Cook and stir until the butter has melted.

4. Serve with fish, sprinkle with almonds with the butter spooned over the fish.

Nutrition Facts Per Serving

Calories 269, Total Fat 19g, Saturated Fat 8g, Total Carbs 2g, Net Carbs 1g, Sugar 1g, Fiber 1g, Protein 22g, Sodium 427mg.

Campfire Salmon

5 Ingredients

- 2 5oz salmon fillets
- 1 tbsp butter, melted
- 1 tbsp lemon juice
- 2 tbsp lemon juice
- 2 lemon wedges

What you' ll need from the store cupboard:

- 1 tbsp minced fresh basil
- ⅛ tsp salt
- ⅛ tsp pepper

Instructions:

1. Place each fillet, skin side on a 12-inch square piece of heavy-duty foil.

2. Mix melted butter, basil, lemon juice, salt and pepper in a bowl. Drizzle over the salmon and seal the foil packets tightly. Fold foil around fish, sealing tightly.

3. Cook on a campfire or in a covered grill for 10-15 minutes.

4. Serve the fish in foil packets on serving plates with lemon wedges.

Nutrition Facts Per Serving

Calories 274, Total Fat 19g, Saturated Fat 6g, Total Carbs 1g, Net Carbs 1g, Sugar 0g, Fiber 0g, Protein 24g, Sodium 264mg

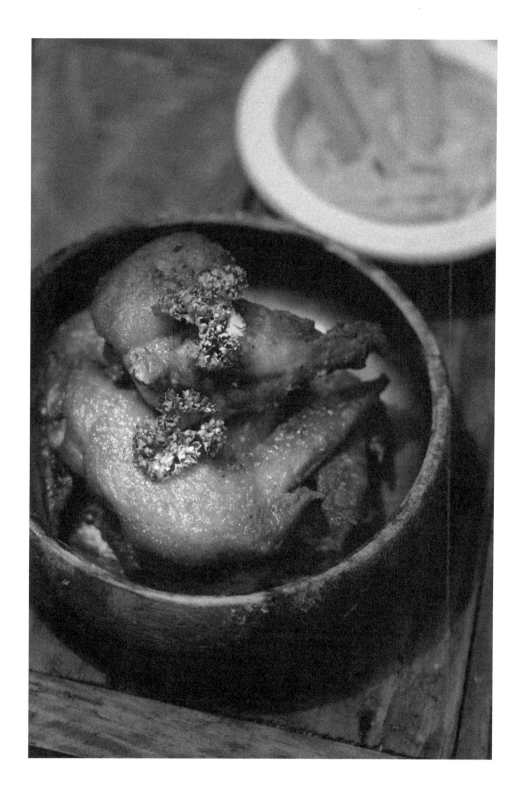

Turkey & Coconut Curry

Prep time: 5 minutes, cook time: 20 minutes; Serves 8

5 Ingredients

- 1½ cups scallions, chopped
- 1 14oz light coconut milk
- ⅔ cup fresh baby spinach, washed and dried

- 4 cup cooked turkey, roughly chopped
- ¼ cup fresh cilantro for garnish

What you' ll need from the store cupboard:

- ¼ cup garlic-infused olive oil
- 1 14oz can diced tomatoes
- 2 tbsp fresh ginger, grated
- 2 tsp ground coriander

- ½ tsp turmeric
- ⅛ tsp cayenne
- 2 tsp ground cumin
- Salt & freshly ground black pepper

Instructions:

1. Heat the oil in a large saucepan and fry 1 cup of the scallion greens for about 3 minutes.

2. Add ginger, cumin, coriander, turmeric, and cayenne and fry slowly to allow the spices to become fragrant.

3. Stir in the tomatoes and the coconut milk. Turn the heat up and bring to a boil, stirring to combine well.

4. Reduce the heat and simmer for a further 5 minutes.

5. Add the spinach and turkey. Heat until the turkey has cooked through and the spinach has wilted.

6. Taste and adjust seasoning if needed. Serve immediately with rice garnished with remaining scallions.

Nutrition Facts Per Serving

Calories 159, Total Fat 11g, Saturated Fat 1g, Total Carbs 10g, Net Carbs 9g, Sugar 1g, Fiber 1g, Protein 9g, Sodium 351mg.

Mozzarella Chicken Fritters

5 Ingredients

- 1lb ground chicken
- ¾ cup mozzarella cheese or soy-based vegan cheese, grated
- ½ tbsp lemon juice
- 1 tsp lemon zest
- 2 tbsp fresh basil, finely chopped

What you ' ll need from the store cupboard:

- 2 large eggs
- ¼ cup mayonnaise
- ¼ cup gluten-free all-purpose flour
- 2 tsp dried chives
- 1 tbsp olive oil
- ¼ tsp salt
- ¼ tsp pepper

Instructions:

1. Place all ingredients except the oil in a bowl and mix well.

2. Heat the oil in a large skillet.

3. Scoop out ¼ cup amounts of measurements and flatten slightly into a fritter shape then drop the fritters into the hot oil. The mixture should make around 8 fritters that you can cook in two batches.

4. Fry the fritters for 3-4 minutes on each side.

5. Serve immediately with potatoes and a salad.

Nutrition Facts Per Serving

Calories 415, Total Fat 27g, Saturated Fat 8g, Total Carbs 11g, Net Carbs 11g, Sugar 2g, Fiber 0g, Protein 31g, Sodium 280mg.

Sweet & Sticky Orange Chicken Wings

Prep time: 5 minutes, cook time: 50 minutes; Serves 5

5 Ingredients

- 2lb chicken wings
- ¼ cup low FODMAP chicken stock
- 1½ tsp orange zest
- ¼ cup freshly squeezed orange juice
- 2 tsp fresh cilantro

What you' ll need from the store cupboard:

- 1 tbsp soy sauce
- 2 tbsp brown sugar
- 1 tbsp vegetable oil

- 2 tsp cornstarch
- 1 tbsp sesame seeds
- Salt and freshly ground pepper

Instructions:

1. Preheat the oven to 400°F.

2. Place the wings in a bowl with the oil and salt and pepper and toss well.

3. Place the wings on a roasting tray and bake for approximately 45 minutes.

4. Toast the sesame seeds in a pan without oil until they begin to brown. Set aside.

5. Dissolve the cornstarch in a little water then place remaining ingredients in a small pan and cook until the sugar has dissolved and the sauce has thickened.

6. Dip the wings in the sauce and sprinkle over the sesame seeds.

7. Garnish with orange zest and fresh cilantro.

Nutrition Facts Per Serving

Calories 334, Total Fat 24g, Saturated Fat 6g, Total Carbs 12g, Net Carbs 10g, Sugar 6g, Fiber 2g, Protein 20g, Sodium 160mg.

Slow Cooker Herby Turkey

Prep time: 10 minutes, cook time: 150 minutes; Serves 20

5 Ingredients

- 5lb whole turkey breast, bone-in, skin-on, split into two pieces

- 1 cup leeks, chopped -green parts only

- 1 tbsp unsalted butter, softened

What you' ll need from the store cupboard:

- 2 tbsp garlic-infused oil

- 1 tsp paprika

- 1 tsp rosemary, crushed

- 2 tbsp brown sugar

- 1 tsp ground sage

- 1 tsp dried thyme

- ½ tsp freshly ground black pepper

Instructions:

1. Scatter the leek and scallion greens in the bottom of your slow cooker.

2. Mix the herbs, spices and salt and pepper with the oil and butter. Use to coat the turkey then place in the slow cooker.

3. Cook the turkey on LOW for 2½ hours.

Nutrition Facts Per Serving

Calories 171, Total Fat 7g, Saturated Fat 1g, Total Carbs 2g, Net Carbs 1g, Sugar 1g, Fiber 1g, Protein 23g, Sodium 175mg.

Chicken Saagwala

5 Ingredients

- 1½lb chicken thighs, boneless and skinless cut into chunks
- 1 cup leek, green tips only, roughly chopped
- 4 cup spinach, roughly chopped
- 2 tsp crushed ginger

What you'll need from the store cupboard:

- 3 tbsp garlic- infused oil
- 1 mild green chilies, deseeded & finely chopped
- 3 tsp ground cumin
- ½ tsp ground turmeric
- ¼ tsp ground cloves
- 1 14oz can crushed tomatoes
- ½ tsp white sugar
- Salt and freshly ground pepper

Instructions:

1. Brown chicken thighs in the garlic olive oil in a large skillet. Set aside.

2. Fry the green leek tips, cumin, cloves, turmeric and crushed ginger in the same pan.

3. Add the spinach leaves and cook for 2 minutes until wilted.

4. Add the crushed tomatoes and mild green chilies and return the chicken to the pan. Simmer gently simmer for approximately 25 minutes.

5. Adjust the seasoning with sugar, salt, and pepper.

Nutrition Facts Per Serving

Calories 375, Total Fat 15g, Saturated Fat 2g, Total Carbs 14g, Net Carbs 11g, Sugar 6g, Fiber 3g, Protein 48g, Sodium 160mg.

Spicy Chicken Drumsticks with Roasted Vegetables

Prep time: 15 minutes, cook time: 45 minutes; Serves 4

5 Ingredients

- 8 chicken drumsticks
- 5 cup potatoes, cut into 1-inch pieces
- 2 cup Japanese pumpkin, or parsnip, cut into 1-inch pieces
- 2 cup broccoli florets
- 2 large carrots, cut into sticks

What you ' ll need from the store cupboard:

- 1½ tbsp maple syrup
- 3 tbsp garlic-infused oil
- ½ tsp ground turmeric
- ½ tsp yellow mustard powder
- 1 tsp ground coriander
- ¼ tsp paprika
- ¼ tsp ground cumin
- ¼ tsp ground cloves
- Salt and freshly ground black pepper

Instructions:

1. Preheat the oven to 350°F.

2. Place the potato and pumpkin pieces in a roasting dish. Drizzle with 1 tablespoon oil and toss to coat. Season with salt and pepper.

3. Mix the remaining oil and maple syrup in a small bowl. Mix the spices in a separate small bowl. Dip the drumsticks in the oil mixture and place in the roasting pan with vegetables. Then sprinkle over the spice mixture.

4. Bake for approximately 45 minutes.

5. Cook the carrots and broccoli by boiling until tender and serve with chicken and roasted vegetables.

Nutrition Facts Per Serving

Calories 555, Total Fat 24g, Saturated Fat 5g, Total Carbs 53g, Net Carbs 43g, Sugar 13g, Fiber 10g, Protein 34g, Sodium 120mg.

Peanut Chicken Satay

5 Ingredients

- 2lbs chicken thighs, skinless, boneless cut into 1-inch wide strips
- 1 tbsp peanut butter

- 2 tbsp dry-roasted peanuts, finely chopped
- ¼ cup hot water

What you' ll need from the store cupboard:

- 5 tbsp garlic-infused oil
- 4 ½ tsp fresh ginger, grated
- 4 tsp turmeric
- 2 tsp Kosher salt
- ¼ cup rice vinegar
- ¼ cup low-sodium soy sauce

- 2 tbsp sugar
- 2 teaspoons peeled & grated fresh ginger
- ½ teaspoon turmeric
- ¼ tsp red pepper flakes
- Bamboo skewers or thin metal skewers

Instructions:

1. Make the marinade by whisking the sugar, 3 tablespoons garlic-infused 0il, 1 teaspoon of ginger, turmeric and 1 teaspoon of salt in a large bowl. Add the chicken and toss well to coat. Allow to marinate for about 30 minutes.

2. Make the satay sauce by whisking together the hot water and peanut butter until smooth in a bowl. Whisk in vinegar, soy sauce, sugar, turmeric and remaining garlic-infused oil, and turmeric. Set aside half of the sauce for dipping later.

3. Thread the chicken onto skewers, discarding the marinade. Place on a grill pan.

4. Grill the chicken for around 7 to 8 minutes brushing all the time with the reserved satay sauce.

5. Serve the chicken satay with the dipping sauce.

Nutrition Facts Per Serving

Calories 228, Total Fat 12g, Saturated Fat 1g, Total Carbs 10g, Net Carbs 9g, Sugar 9g, Fiber 1g, Protein 19g, Sodium 671mg.

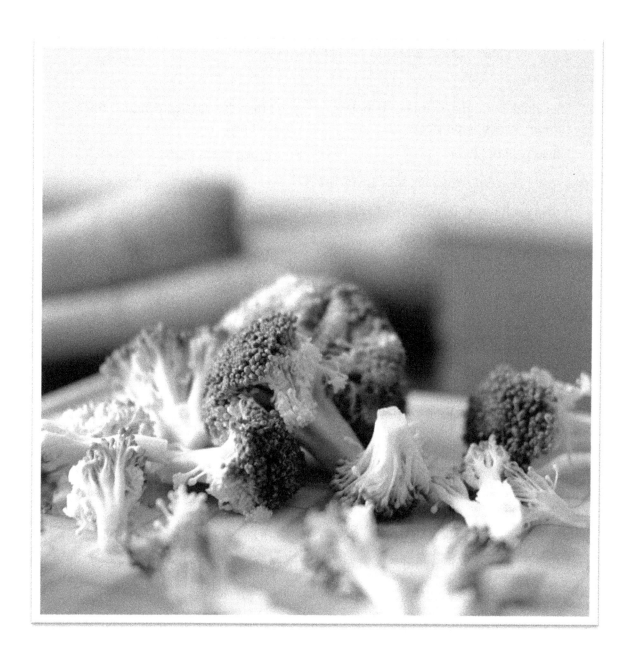

Crispy Roasted Potatoes

Prep time: 10 minutes, cook time: 60 minutes; Serves 4

5 Ingredients

- 4 tbsp dairy-free spread, melted
- 5 cup potatoes, sliced into ⅛ inch thick slices
- 1½ tsp fresh thyme

What you'll need from the store cupboard

- ¼ tsp salt
- ⅛ tsp dried chili flakes
- Black pepper

Instructions:

1. Preheat the oven to 375°F.

2. Brush the bottom of a 10-inch oven-proof skillet with 1 tablespoon of the spread.

3. Stack the potato pieces in the frypan in an upright position.

4. Brush the remaining potatoes with the remaining spread and sprinkle with fresh thyme salt and black pepper, and chili flakes.

5. Place in the oven and bake for approximately 1 hour.

Nutrition Facts Per Serving

Calories 257, Total Fat 11g, Saturated Fat 2g, Total Carbs 35g, Net Carbs 31g, Sugar 2g, Fiber 4g, Protein 4g, Sodium 120mg.

Bacon & Egg Salad

5 Ingredients

- 1 cup baby spinach

- 4oz bacon strips, cut into small strips

- 1 small cucumber, peeled and thinly sliced

- 2 medium tomato, cut into small pieces

- 1 cup baby spinach

What you' ll need from the store cupboard:

- 2 large eggs, hard-boiled

- 4 tbsp mayonnaise

- 1 tsp garlic-infused oil

- Freshly ground black pepper

Instructions:

1. Fry the bacon in a skillet until crispy.

2. Mix the mayonnaise and garlic-infused oil in a small bowl until smooth. Season with black pepper.

3. Place the garlic-infused mayonnaise into mason jars.

4. Top with the salad then the bacon and egg. Chill until ready to serve.

Nutrition Facts Per Serving

Calories 429, Total Fat 35g, Saturated Fat 10g, Total Carbs 13g, Net Carbs 10g, Sugar 7g, Fiber 3g, Protein 17g, Sodium 280mg.

Potato & Egg Salad

5 Ingredients

- 5 cup potatoes, cut into small pieces
- 1 small cucumber, peeled and cut into small strips
- 1 cup green beans, cut into small pieces
- 1 red bell pepper,
- 3 tbsp green scallions, green tips only and finely chopped

What you'll need from the store cupboard:

- 4 large egg, hard-boiled and cut into quarters
- 1 tbsp lemon juice
- 3 tbsp fresh chives
- ⅓ cup mayonnaise
- 1 tbsp wholegrain mustard
- Freshly ground black pepper

Instructions:

1. Place the potatoes in a large saucepan and boil for 15 minutes.

2. Add the green beans to the potatoes for the last 5 minutes of cooking time. When vegetables are tender, drain and set aside to cool.

3. Make the dressing by mixing the wholegrain mustard, mayonnaise, and lemon juice in a small bowl. Season with black pepper.

4. In a large bowl mix all ingredients until well combined. Add more pepper if desired.

Nutrition Facts Per Serving

Calories 327, Total Fat 11g, Saturated Fat 3g, Total Carbs 44g, Net Carbs 38g, Sugar 6g, Fiber 6g, Protein 14g, Sodium 160mg.

Mustard Salmon Jar Salad

5 Ingredients

- 2 oz fresh salmon fillets
- 1 cup lettuce, shredded
- ½ red bell peppers, diced
- ¼ cup cucumber, diced
- 2 tbsp avocado, diced

What you' ll need from the store cupboard:

- 1 tbsp lemon juice
- 1 tbsp olive oil
- ½ tsp Dijon mustard
- 1 tsp vegetable oil
- Freshly ground black pepper

Instructions:

1. Preheat the oven to 400ºF.

2. Place the salmon fillet in a small ovenproof dish. Drizzle with vegetable oil and season with salt and pepper. Bake for approximately 12 minutes until the salmon is cooked. Set aside to cool.

3. Mix the olive oil, mustard, and lemon juice in a small bowl to make a dressing.

4. Toss the avocado in a few drops of lemon juice and combine with salad ingredients.

5. Shred the cooled salmon and mix into the salad.

6. Pile into mason jars and chill until serving.

Nutrition Facts Per Serving

Calories 310, Total Fat 22g, Saturated Fat 3g, Total Carbs 12g, Net Carbs 7g, Sugar 5g, Fiber 5g, Protein 17g, Sodium 40mg

Ginger Roasted Vegetables

Prep time: 15 minutes, cook time: 45 minutes; Serves 6

5 Ingredients

- 12oz carrots, cut into chunks

- 12oz sweet potato, cut into chunks

- 12 oz Japanese pumpkin, Kabocha squash or parsnip, cut into chunks

- 5 cup potatoes, cut into chunks

- 2 red bell peppers, cut into chunks

What you' ll need from the store cupboard:

- 12oz drained canned beetroot, cut into chunks

- 4 tbsp olive oil

- 1½ tbsp fresh ginger, crushed

- 1 tbsp maple syrup

- Salt and freshly ground pepper

Instructions:

1. Preheat the oven to 375°F.

2. Line a roasting tray with parchment paper

2. Place the vegetables in the roasting tray in a single layer and toss with a small amount of olive oil. Season with salt and pepper.

4. Mix the olive oil, crushed ginger and maple syrup in a small bowl.

5. Baste the vegetable and place in the oven.

6. Roast the vegetables for approximately 45 minutes, basting frequently with marinade.

Nutrition Facts Per Serving

Calories 316, Total Fat 10g, Saturated Fat 2g, Total Carbs 53g, Net Carbs 43g, Sugar 16g, Fiber 10g, Protein 6g, Sodium 80mg

Cheesy Broccoli & Zucchini Fritters

5 Ingredients

- 2 cup broccoli florets, steamed
- 1 cup zucchini, grated
- ½ cup Colby, Cheddar or soy-based vegan cheese, grated
- 2 tsp fresh lime juice & ½ tsp lime zest
- 3 tbsp low FODMAP milk

What you' ll need from the store cupboard:

- ½ cup gluten-free all-purpose flour
- ¼ tsp salt
- ¼ tsp black pepper

- 1 egg, beaten
- 2 tbsp garlic-infused oil
- ¼ cup mayonnaise

Instructions:

1. Mash the steamed broccoli. Set aside.

2. Whisk together the egg, milk, and 1 tablespoon of garlic-infused oil in a small bowl.

3. Mix in the flour, salt, and black pepper until thick and smooth.

4. Now add the steamed broccoli, zucchini, and cheese.

5. Heat remaining oil in a large skillet. Add quarter cup measures of the fritters and flatten own with a spatula.

6. Cook the fritters for 3-4 minutes each side.

7. Mix the lime juice and zest with the mayonnaise. Serve alongside the fritters.

Nutrition Facts Per Serving

Calories 310, Total Fat 17g, Saturated Fat 6g, Total Carbs 28g, Net Carbs 26g, Sugar 4g, Fiber 2g, Protein 11g, Sodium 200mg

Bacon, Sweet Potato & Kale Hash

5 Ingredients

- 1 sweet potato, peeled and diced into ¼ -inch cubes

- 3 rashers bacon,

- 1 cup kale, chopped with stalks removed

- 1 bell pepper, diced

What you ' ll need from the store cupboard:

- 3 eggs

- 1 tbsp vegetable oil

- Salt and freshly ground pepper to taste

Instructions:

1. Preheat your oven to 400°F.

2. Fry the bacon until crisp in a large ovenproof skillet. Remove from the pan and set aside.

3. Arrange the sweet potato in the skillet and cook undisturbed until brown on one side.

4. Flip the sweet potato cubes over and brown on the other side.

5. Add the kale and bell peppers and stir to soften the vegetables. Season with salt and pepper.

6. Make wells in the mixture and crack in the eggs.

7. Transfer the skillet to the oven and cook for approximately 10 minutes depending on how you like your eggs.

8. Serve with bacon crumbled over the top.

Nutrition Facts Per Serving

Calories 161, Total Fat 9g, Saturated Fat 2g, Total Carbs 14g, Net Carbs 10g, Sugar 5g, Fiber 4g, Protein 9g, Sodium 181mg

Maple, Orange & Thyme Glazed Baby Carrots

5 Ingredients

- 2 cup baby carrots, trimmed and scrubbed
- 2½ tbsp butter, salted
- ½ cup freshly squeezed orange juice
- 1 tsp orange zest
- 1 tbsp thyme, chopped

What you' ll need from the store cupboard:

- ⅓ cup maple syrup
- ½ tsp salt
- ½ tsp black pepper
- 1 tbsp mustard

Instructions:

1. Melt the butter in a large non-stick skillet pan with a close-fitting lid.

2. Add carrots, maple syrup, orange juice, zest, and the salt and pepper.

3. Bring to the boil and cover with the lid. Reduce the heat and cook for about 4 minutes.

4. Uncover and cook for a further 15 minutes.

5. Serve garnished with fresh thyme.

Nutrition Facts Per Serving

Calories 185, Total Fat 10g, Saturated Fat 7g, Total Carbs 22g, Net Carbs 19g, Sugar 11g, Fiber 3g, Protein 1g, Sodium 477mg, 7 Beef lamb and pork

Glazed Ham

5 Ingredients

- 1 16lb ham on the bone
- ⅓ cup freshly squeezed orange juice

What you' ll need from the store cupboard:

- ⅓ cup brown sugar
- ⅓ cup maple syrup
- 1 tbsp Dijon mustard
- 30 whole cloves

Instructions:

1. Preheat the oven to 300°F.

2. Line a large baking tray with two layers of baking paper.

3. Place the ham in the baking tray and place in the oven for 10 minutes to warm the skin.

4. Whisk together the maple syrup, brown sugar, orange juice, and dijon mustard in a small bowl.

5. Remove the ham from the oven and increase the oven temperature to 340°F.

6. Make a cut around the ham using a sharp knife then use your fingers to peel away the rind and fat.

7. Score the ham in a diamond pattern, and stud the centers of the diamonds with cloves. Baste with glaze and place into the oven.

8. Bake for approximately 4 hours basting every half hour.

Nutrition Facts Per Serving

Calories 495, Total Fat 18g, Saturated Fat 6g, Total Carbs 6g, Net Carbs 6g, Sugar 5g, Fiber 0g, Protein 72g, Sodium 2000mg

Beef Burgers with BBQ Sauce

5 Ingredients

- 1lb lean ground beef
- ¼ cup green scallions, green tips only, finely chopped
- ¼ cup gluten-free breadcrumbs
- 3 medium carrots, peeled & cut into chunks

What you'll need from the store cupboard:

- ½ tsp dried thyme
- 1 tsp dried oregano
- 1 tsp dried basil
- 1 tbsp Worcestershire sauce

- Salt & pepper
- 1½ tsp vegetable oil
- Salt & freshly ground black pepper
- 1 large egg, lightly beaten

Instructions:

1. Preheat the oven to 410°F.

2. Place the carrots into a roasting tray and toss with oil. Bake for approximately 30 minutes.

3. In a large bowl, mix the lean ground beef, scallions tips, breadcrumbs, dried herbs, Worcestershire sauce, beaten egg, and salt and pepper.

4. Divide the mixture evenly into 8 patties.

5. Fry the patties for 7 minutes each side.

4. Serve the burgers on toasted the gluten-free buns if desired with shredded lettuce, tomatoes, and cucumber.

Nutrition Facts Per Serving

Calories 613, Total Fat 23g, Saturated Fat 6g, Total Carbs 62g, Net Carbs 49g, Sugar 20g, Fiber 13g, Protein 40g, Sodium 360mg

Spaghetti Bolognese

5 Ingredients

- 1lb lean ground beef
- ½ cup leek, green tips only, thinly sliced
- 4 cup baby spinach, roughly chopped
- 1 cup green beans, cut into small pieces
- 2 large carrots, peeled & cut into sticks

What you' ll need from the store cupboard:

- 1 tbsp olive oil
- 3 tbsp tomato paste
- 1 tsp dried oregano
- 1 tsp dried basil

- ½ tsp dried thyme
- 12oz gluten-free spaghetti
- 1 14oz can crushed tomatoes
- Salt & freshly ground pepper

Instructions:

1. Cook the beef until browned in a large skillet.

2. Add canned tomatoes, tomato paste, leek tips, baby spinach, and herbs and allow to simmer for 20 minutes. Add salt and pepper to taste.

4. Cook the pasta according to the instructions on the packet.

5. Cook green beans and carrots in boiling water until tender.

6. Serve the bolognese on a bed of spaghetti with the cheese on top and a side of vegetables.

Nutrition Facts Per Serving

Calories 642, Total Fat 19g, Saturated Fat 7g, Total Carbs 82g, Net Carbs 67g, Sugar 11g, Fiber 15g, Protein 40g, Sodium 200mg

Espresso Ribeye

5 Ingredients

- 1 2lb bone-in rib-eye steak, about 1½ inches thick
- 1 tbsp salted butter

What you'll need from the store cupboard:

- 1½ tbsp vegetable oil
- 1½ tsp flaky sea salt
- 1 tsp black pepper
- ⅓ cup instant espresso granules
- 2 tsp ancho chili powder

Instructions:

1. Preheat the oven to 450°F.

2. Rub both sides of the steak with ½ tablespoon of the oil, and season with salt and pepper.

3. Rub both sides of the steak with the espresso granules and chili powder. Set aside for 30 minutes.

4. Place an ovenproof skillet in the oven until hot for 10 minutes.

5. Remove the hot skillet from the oven and add the remaining oil to the pan.

6. Place the steak in the skillet and leave to cook for 3 minutes.

7. Flip the steak and cook, undisturbed, again for a further 3 minutes.

8. Use tongs to hold the edges of the steak to the pan. Cook for an additional 6 minutes this way.

9. Place the steak in the skillet in the oven for 6 to 8 minutes for medium-rare.

10. Remove the steak from the skillet; top with the butter, and let rest for 10 minutes before serving.

Nutrition Facts Per Serving

Calories 552, Total Fat 46g, Saturated Fat 2g, Total Carbs 3g, Net Carbs 2g, Sugar 1g, Fiber 1g, Protein 8g, Sodium 461mg

Sweet Potato & Lamb Fritters with Salad

5 Ingredients

- 10oz sweet potato, peeled & diced

- 10oz potato, peeled & diced

- 1lb lean ground lamb

- 1 cup green scallions, green tips only, finely chopped

- 1 cup fresh cilantro, chopped

What you' ll need from the store cupboard:

- 1 tbsp garlic-infused oil

- 1 tbsp crushed ginger

- 2 tsp soy sauce

- 1 tbsp oyster sauce

Instructions:

1. Preheat the oven to 350ºF.

2. Boil the sweet potatoes and potatoes until tender. Then roughly mash with a fork. Set aside.

3. Heat the oil in a large skillet and fry the lamb.

4. Add ginger, spring onion tips, soy sauce, oyster sauce, and fresh cilantro.

5. Mix the lamb with the potato mixture in a large bowl.

6. Scoop out quarter cup measures of mixture and shape into fritters. Place the fritters on a baking pan lined with parchment paper.

7. Place in the oven and bake for 10 minutes each side, until golden brown.

8. Serve with a salad made of lettuce, grated carrot, tomatoes, and cucumbers.

Nutrition Facts Per Serving

Calories 465, Total Fat 27g, Saturated Fat 12g, Total Carbs 33g, Net Carbs 27g, Sugar 8g, Fiber 6g, Protein 24g, Sodium 160mg

Pork Loin with Maple Mustard Sauce

5 Ingredients

- 1 3lb pork loin
- ½ tsp smoked paprika

What you' ll need from the store cupboard:

- 4 tbsp maple syrup
- 4 tbsp wholegrain mustard
- Salt and freshly ground black pepper
- 1 teaspoon dry rosemary, crushed

Instructions:

1. Preheat oven to 350°F.

2. Mix maple syrup and mustard in a small bowl.

3. Season the pork loin with salt and pepper. Sprinkle with rosemary and paprika.

4. Place pork loin in roasting pan and brush with maple mustard sauce.

5. Roast for about 1 hour, basting with extra sauce halfway through cooking.

Nutrition Facts Per Serving

Calories 271, Total Fat 17g, Saturated Fat 1g, Total Carbs 7g, Net Carbs 6g, Sugar 1g, Fiber 1g, Protein 22g, Sodium 1mg

Beef Stroganoff

5 Ingredients

- 1lb sirloin, cut into ¼ inch thick, 1 inch wide and 2 inch long strips
- 3 cup oyster mushrooms, coarsely chopped
- ½ cup dry sherry
- ½ cup lactose-free sour cream
- ⅓ cup scallions, green parts only, finely chopped

What you' ll need from the store cupboard:

- 2 tsp Dijon mustard
- 4 tbsp oil
- 2 tbsp cornstarch
- 12oz gluten-free tagliatelle
- 2 cup low FODMAP beef stock
- ¼ tsp sweet paprika
- Salt and freshly ground black pepper

Instructions:

1. Season the meat with salt and pepper.

2. Heat 1 tablespoon of oil in a large skillet and cook the beef. Set aside.

3. Heat 2 tablespoons of oil and fry leeks and scallions for 2 minutes.

4. Add mushrooms and cook for 3 more minutes.

5. Add the beef stock and sherry blended with cornstarch and cook until the sauce has thickened. Stir in 1 tablespoon dill and ¼ teaspoon paprika.

6. Return the meat to the pan and cook until beef is hot.

7. Cook pasta until al dente and toss in remaining oil.

8. Serve the stroganoff with the pasta garnished with the remaining dill and paprika.

Nutrition Facts Per Serving

Calories 607, Total Fat 27g, Saturated Fat 1g, Total Carbs 52g, Net Carbs 50g, Sugar 2g, Fiber 2g, Protein 34g, Sodium 166mg

Bacon-Wrapped Pork Loin with Brown Sugar & Marmalade

Prep time: 5 minutes, cook time: 35 minutes; Serves 4

5 Ingredients

- 1 1½lb pork loin, patted dry
- ½ tsp paprika
- 4 slices meaty bacon
- ¼ cup orange marmalade

What you'll need from the store cupboard:

- 3 tbsp firmly packed light brown sugar
- ¼ tsp thyme
- 2 tsp kosher salt
- ½ tsp freshly ground black pepper
- 1 tbsp garlic-Infused Oil, made with vegctable oil or purchased equivalent
- 2 tbsp Dijon mustard

Instructions:

1. Preheat oven to 350°F/180°C.

2. Mix the brown sugar, thyme, salt, pepper and paprika in a small bowl.

3. Rub the glaze over the pork loin, then wrap bacon around the pork. .

4. Heat oil in a large ovenproof skillet. Sear the tenderloin for 6 minutes on each side.

5. Mix the marmalade and mustard in a small bowl. Brush the tenderloin with the marmalade and place in the oven.

6. Roast for 20 minutes.

7. Transfer to a board and leave to rest covered with foil for 5 minutes.

8. Serve with potatoes and low FODMAP vegetables.

Nutrition Facts Per Serving

Calories 588, Total Fat 36g, Saturated Fat 1g, Total Carbs 20g, Net Carbs 19g, Sugar 18g, Fiber 1g, Protein 43g, Sodium 1256mg

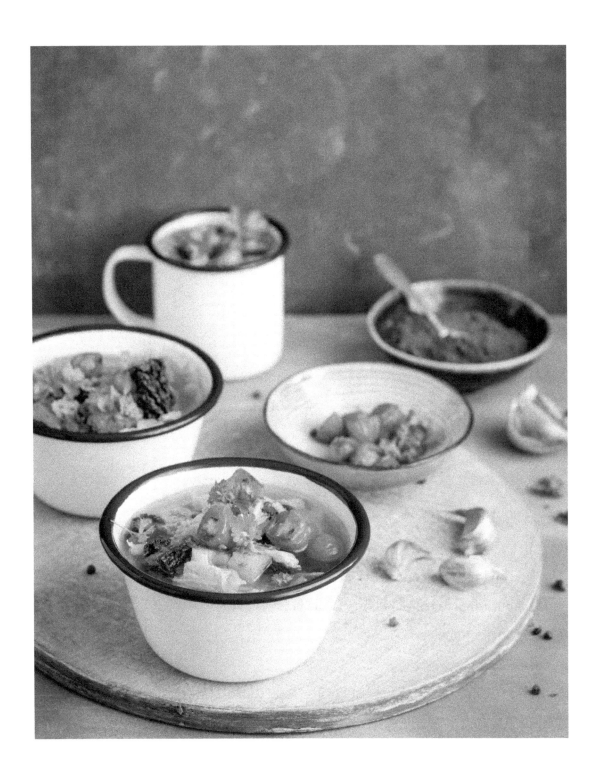

Vegetable & Chickpea Soup

Prep time: 15 minutes, cook time: 25 minutes; Serves 10

5 Ingredients

- 2 cup leek leaves, cut into ½-inch pieces
- 12 cup mixed vegetables, cut into ½ -inch pieces
- 1 14oz tin chickpeas, drained
- ½ bunch silverbeet, chopped
- 1 bunch parsley stalks and leaves, chopped

What you' ll need from the store cupboard:

- ⅓ cup garlic-infused olive oil.
- 1½ quarts water
- 1 28oz diced tomatoes
- 2 tsp salt
- 2 tsp black pepper

Instructions:

1. Heat the oil in a large pan fry the leek leaves.

2. Add all other ingredients and bring to the boil.

3. Simmer for 15 minutes.

Nutrition Facts Per Serving

Calories 185, Total Fat 7g, Saturated Fat 1g, Total Carbs 21g, Net Carbs 12g, Protein 6g, Fiber 9g, Sodium 629mg.

Thai Pumpkin Noodle Soup

5 Ingredients

- 5 cup Japanese pumpkin, peeled, deseeded & cut into cubes
- 1 cup carrot, peeled & cut into cubes
- 2 cup thin rice noodles

- 1 cup green onions/scallions, green tips only, finely chopped
- 1 ½ cup coconut milk

What you' ll need from the store cupboard:

- 1 tsp ground cumin
- 1 tbsp olive oil
- 1 tsp crushed ginger
- 2 tsp Thai fish sauce

- ⅛ tsp dried chilli flakes
- 2 cup low FODMAP chicken stock/vegetable stock
- Salt & freshly ground pepper

Instructions:

1. Preheat the oven to 350°F

2. Place the carrot and pumpkin in a roasting tray and drizzle with oil, toss until well coated. Sprinkle with cumin and season well with salt and pepper.

3. Bake in the oven for 20 to 30 minutes, turning once. Set aside and leave to cool for 10 minutes.

4. Blitz the vegetables in a blender with the stock.

5. Heat a drizzle of olive oil in a large saucepan and fry the spring onion tips for 2 to 3 minutes. Add ginger and cook for a further minute.

6. Add pureed pumpkin, coconut milk, fish sauce, and chili flakes. Allow to simmer over low heat for 10 to 15 minutes.

7. Cook your noodles according to packet directions

8. Before serving add cooked noodles. Garnish with fresh cilantro if desired.

Nutrition Facts Per Serving

Calories 372, Total Fat 16g, Saturated Fat 12g, Total Carbs 53g, Net Carbs 45g, Sugar 8g, Fiber 8g, Protein 8g, Sodium 280mg

Simple Lamb Stew

5 Ingredients

- 1lb lamb leg steaks, cut into cubes
- 2 large carrots, peeled and cut into cubes
- 2 cup potato, peeled and cut into cubes
- 2 cup sweet potato
- 1 cup green beans

What you' ll need from the store cupboard:

- 1 tbsp vegetable oil
- 1 tbsp garlic-infused oil
- 1 cup boiling water
- 4 cup low FODMAP beef stock or chicken stock

- 1 tsp dried oregano
- ½ tsp dried thyme
- Salt & pepper

Instructions:

1. Grease the slow cooker dish with cooking oil and set to LOW.

2. Brown the lamb for 4 to 5 minutes in a large skillet.

3. Add the lamb, green leek tips, carrot, potato, oil, oregano, thyme, stock, black pepper, and boiling water to the slow cooker.

4. Leave the slow cooker to cook on LOW for 8 to 10 hours.

5. Boil the green beans for 2 to 3 minutes until tender. Stir through the stew.

6. Serve the stew with toasted gluten-free bread and garnish with fresh parsley.

Nutrition Facts Per Serving

Calories 703, Total Fat 36g, Saturated Fat 13g, Total Carbs 64g, Net Carbs 55g, Sugar 12g, Fiber 9g, Protein 33g, Sodium 600mg

Beef & Leek Stew

5 Ingredients

- 1lb beef chuck steak, cut into 1-inch cubes
- 1 14oz can chopped tomatoes
- 2 large carrots, peeled & roughly chopped
- ¾ cup leek, green tips only, roughly sliced
- 2 tsp lemon juice

What you' ll need from the store cupboard:

- 1 tbsp olive oil
- 1 tbsp garlic infused oil
- 3 tbsp tomato paste
- 1 cup low FODMAP chicken stock
- 1 tsp dried oregano
- 2 bay leaves
- 1 tsp dried basil
- 2 tsp cornstarch, dissolved in 2 tbsp cold water
- Salt & freshly ground pepper

Instructions:

1. Rub beef with olive oil and season with salt and pepper.

2. Heat garlic-infused oil in a large skillet and brown beef.

3. Add the beef, tomatoes, tomato paste, green leek tips, chopped carrots, oregano, bay leaf, basil, and salt and pepper to a slow cooker.

4. Cook on LOW for 9 hours.

5. Add the cornstarch to the stew and the lemon juice.

6. Allow to thicken and serve with toasted gluten-free bread.

Nutrition Facts Per Serving

Calories 515, Total Fat 18g, Saturated Fat 4g, Total Carbs 52g, Net Carbs 46g, Sugar 13g, Fiber 6g, Protein 41g, Sodium 400mg

Carrot & Fennel Soup

5 Ingredients

- 2 large carrots, peeled and cut into small pieces
- 2 cup potatoes, peeled and cut into small pieces

- 1 cup sweet potatoes, peeled and cut into small pieces
- ½ cup leek, green tips only, thinly sliced
- ½ cup low FODMAP milk

What you' ll need from the store cupboard:

- 1 tbsp garlic-infused oil
- 1 tbsp olive oil
- 3 cup low FODMAP chicken stock/vegetable stock

- 1 tbsp olive oil
- 2 tsp fennel seeds
- Salt & freshly ground black pepper

Instructions:

1. Heat the garlic-infused oil and olive oil in a large saucepan and fry the leek tips for a few minutes

2. Add potatoes, carrots, and sweet potato to the pan, and cook over low heat for a further 5 minutes.

3. Add the stock to the saucepan and bring to the boil. Allow the soup to cook on a rolling boil for around 15 minutes or until vegetables are tender.

4. Melt the dairy-free spread in a frying pan. Fry the fennel seeds for 1 minute, then add the fresh cilantro and cook for a further minute.

5. Add the fresh cilantro and fennel seed mixture to the soup.

6. Blitz the soup in batches in a blender.

7. Return the soup to the pan and add the milk.

8. Heat soup through and serve with fresh cilantro and a side of toasted low FODMAP bread.

Nutrition Facts Per Serving

Calories 416, Total Fat 12g, Saturated Fat 2g, Total Carbs 67g, Net Carbs 60g, Sugar 11g, Fiber 7g, Protein 11g, Sodium 520mg

Chicken & Leek Soup

Prep time: 20 minutes, cook time: 7 hours; Serves 4

5 Ingredients

- 1lb chicken breast fillets
- 2 large carrots, peeled & chopped
- 2 cup Japanese pumpkin, Kabocha squash or parsnip
- ½ cup leek, green tips only
- 3 tbsp fresh parsley, finely chopped

What you' ll need from the store cupboard:

- 2 tbsp garlic-infused oil
- 4 cup low FODMAP chicken stock
- ½ tsp dried thyme
- ½ tsp dried rosemary
- 2 dried bay leaf
- 1 tbsp lemon juice
- Salt & freshly ground black pepper

Instructions:

1. Spray a slow cooker dish with oil.

2. Place chicken breasts, vegetables and herbs in the slow cooker.

3. Cover ingredients low FODMAP chicken stock and season with salt & pepper.

4. Cook on LOW for 7 hours.

5. Before serving shred the chicken breasts.

6. Serve with toasted gluten-free bread and a sprinkle of fresh parsley.

Nutrition Facts Per Serving

Calories 474, Total Fat 14g, Saturated Fat 2g, Total Carbs 45g, Net Carbs 39g, Sugar 9g, Fiber 6g, Protein 43g, Sodium 600mg

Sweet Red Pepper Soup

5 Ingredients

- 2 red bell pepper, deseeded & cut into strips
- 2 large carrots, peeled & chopped
- 2 medium parsnips, peeled & chopped
- 3 tbsp fresh parsley

What you' ll need from the store cupboard:

- 1 tbsp vegetable oil
- 1 14oz can crushed tomatoes
- 1 tbsp garlic-infused oil
- 2 tsp paprika
- 4 cup low FODMAP chicken stock/vegetable stock
- Salt & freshly ground pepper

Instructions:

1.Preheat the oven to 400°F

2. Place the vegetables in a roasting tray. Drizzle with oil and season with salt and pepper. Toss to coat and roast for 20 to 25 minutes.

3. Blitz the roasted vegetables in a blender with the stock and tomatoes.

4. Transfer the soup to a large saucepan. Heat through and serve with toasted gluten-free bread and a sprinkle of fresh parsley.

Nutrition Facts Per Serving

Calories 366, Total Fat 10g, Saturated Fat 1g, Total Carbs 61g, Net Carbs 51g, Sugar 17g, Fiber 10g, Protein 11g, Sodium 680mg

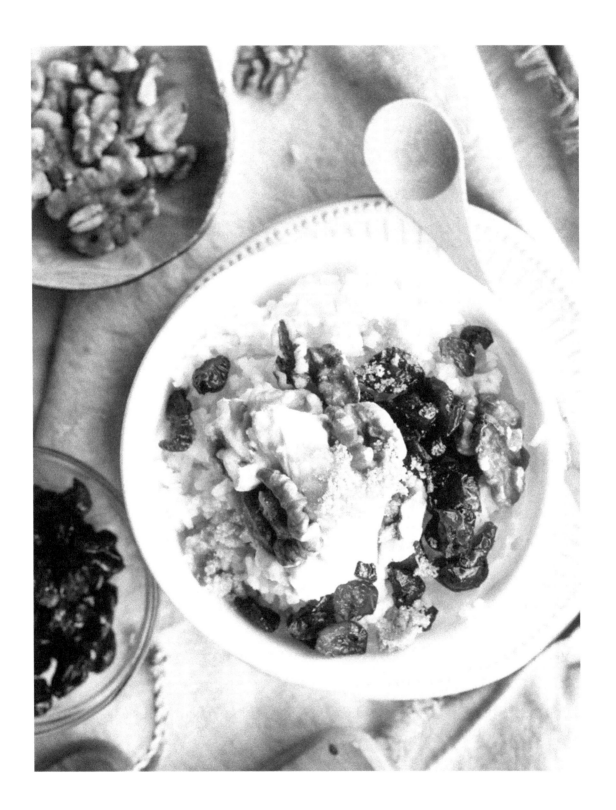

Vegetable Fried Rice

Prep time: 10 minutes, cook time: 10 minutes; Serves 4

5 Ingredients

- ½ cup scallions, green tips only, finely sliced
- 3 medium carrots, diced
- 3 large eggs, beaten
- 4 cups cooked rice, white or brown
- 12 sugar snap peas, diagonally sliced crosswise into thirds

What you' ll need from the store cupboard:

- 2 tbsp garlic-Infused oil
- ¼ cup low FODMAP oyster sauce
- 1 tbsp toasted sesame oil
- Low FODMAP hot sauce

Instructions:

1. Heat oil in a wok and stir-fry scallions for 30 seconds.

2. Add carrots and snap peas and stir-fry for 1 minute.

3. Add eggs for just a few seconds then add rice. Use a spatula to cut the eggs through the rice.

4. Add oyster sauce, toasted sesame oil, hot sauce. Stir well and serve immediately.

Nutrition Facts Per Serving

Calories 425, Total Fat 14g, Saturated Fat 0g, Total Carbs 62g, Net Carbs 62g, Sugar 2g, Fiber 1g, Protein 10g, Sodium 45mg.

Easy Low FODMAP Salmon Fried Rice

5 Ingredients

- 1 red bell peppers, sliced

- 1 large carrot, peeled & grated

- ½ cup green beans, cut into pieces

- 1 8oz can pink salmon

- ½ cup green scallions, green tips only, finely sliced

What you' ll need from the store cupboard:

- 1 tbsp sesame oil

- 1 tbsp garlic-infused oil

- 2 tsp crushed ginger

- 2 large eggs

- 2 cup cooked long-grain white rice

- 2 tsp Thai fish sauce

- 2 tbsp soy sauce

Instructions:

1. Heat sesame oil and garlic-infused oil in a wok.

2. Fry the crushed ginger and scallions for 1 to 2 minutes.

3. Add the red bell pepper and fry for 1 minute. Add the grated carrots, green beans, and tinned salmon to the frypan and cook for 2 minutes.

4. Add the fish sauce and crack the eggs into the wok. Stir the egg through the vegetables until cooked.

5. Add the rice and soy sauce. Heat through and serve immediately.

Nutrition Facts Per Serving

Calories 522, Total Fat 18g, Saturated Fat 3g, Total Carbs 61g, Net Carbs 58g, Sugar 4g, Fiber 3g, Protein 29g, Sodium 560mg

Pumpkin & Carrot Risotto

Prep time: 25 minutes, cook time: 35 minutes; Serves 4

5 Ingredients

- 9oz Japanese pumpkin, cut into ½-inch pieces
- ½ cup leek, green tips only
- 4 cup spinach, shredded
- 2½ tbsp lemon juice & 2 tsp lemon zest
- 2 large carrots, cut into ½-inch pieces

What you'll need from the store cupboard:

- 2 tbsp olive oil
- 1 tbsp garlic-infused oil
- 4 cups low FODMAP chicken stock/vegetable stock
- 1½ cup risotto rice
- Salt & freshly ground black pepper

Instructions:

1. Preheat the oven to 400ºF.

2. Place pumpkin & carrot in an oven dish, drizzle with olive oil and season with salt and pepper.

3. Bake for 20 to 25 minutes.

4. .Melt the dairy-free spread in a large saucepan with garlic-infused oil for two minutes. Add the rice, stir through the mixture for about 1 minute.

5. Add stock, half a cup at a time until the liquid has absorbed into the rice each time.

6. Keep adding the stock, half a cup at a time until all the stock has been added and the rice has cooked.

7. When the rice is cooked, add the roasted vegetables, shredded spinach, lemon juice, and lemon zest. Season with salt and pepper.

8. Serve garnished with fresh cilantro and Parmesan cheese.

Nutrition Facts Per Serving

Calories 501, Total Fat 15g, Saturated Fat 4g, Total Carbs 80g, Net Carbs 75g, Sugar 7g, Fiber 5g, Protein 12g, Sodium 560mg

Spaghetti all' Amatriciana

5 Ingredients

- 4oz pancetta, cut into small strips
- ¼ cup dry white wine
- ¼ cup grated Pecorino Romano

What you' ll need from the store cupboard:

- 1 tbsp extra virgin garlic-infused olive oil
- 1 28oz can diced tomatoes
- 1lb gluten-free spaghetti
- ½ tsp red pepper flakes
- Freshly ground black pepper

Instructions:

1. Heat the oil in a large skillet over medium heat. Add pancetta and sauté for 4 minutes.

2. Add pepper flakes, black pepper and wine. Continue to cook until the liquid has reduced.

3. Add tomatoes and simmer for 20 minutes

4. Cook pasta until just firmer than al dente. Drain pasta, reserving 1 cup of pasta cooking water.

5. Add drained pasta to the sauce. Add the reserved water a few tablespoons at a time until the sauce until sauce comes together with pasta is coated evenly and well.

6. Add cheese and serve immediately.

Nutrition Facts Per Serving

Calories 327, Total Fat 12g, Saturated Fat 1g, Total Carbs 46g, Net Carbs 43g, Sugar 3g, Fiber 3g, Protein 8g, Sodium 149mg

Tuna & Sun-Dried Tomato Rigatoni

5 Ingredients

- ⅓ cup scallions, green parts only, finely chopped
- ¼ cup grated Parmesan cheese
- 2 5oz cans tuna, drained well
- 2 medium tomatoes, cored and halved crosswise
- ⅓ cup fresh flat-leaf parsley, finely chopped

What you'll need from the store cupboard:

- 2 tbsp garlic-infused olive oil
- 1 tbsp red wine vinegar
- 12oz low FODMAP gluten-free rigatoni
- ¾oz oil-packed sun-dried tomatoes, drained and finely chopped
- Pinch of red pepper flakes
- Salt and freshly ground black pepper

Instructions:

1. Heat a large skillet and add scallion greens and sun-dried tomatoes and fry for 1 minute.

2. Add the fresh tomatoes, tuna, vinegar, and red pepper flakes. Sauté around for 2 minutes.

3. Cook the pasta until al dente and add to the pan.

3. Add half of the parsley and Parmesan and toss until cheese has melted.

4. Add a little of the reserved pasta water if the sauce needs some liquid.

5. Season with salt and pepper as desired. Serve topped with remaining Parmesan and parsley.

Nutrition Facts Per Serving

Calories 355, Total Fat 10g, Saturated Fat 1g, Total Carbs 45g, Net Carbs 42g, Sugar 1g, Fiber 3g, Protein 24g, Sodium 64mg

Pasta Salad with Chickpeas & Feta

Prep time: 10 minutes, cook time: 10 minutes; Serves 8

5 Ingredients

- ½ cup cherry or grape tomatoes, halved
- ¼ cup scallions, green parts only, finely chopped
- 4 small Persian style cucumbers, cut into ½-inch rounds
- 1 red or orange bell pepper, cut into bite-sized pieces
- 1lb feta, drained and cubed

What you'll need from the store cupboard:

- ¼ cup extra-virgin olive oil
- ¼ cup white wine vinegar or apple cider vinegar
- 1 tbsp Dijon mustard
- Kosher salt
- Freshly ground black pepper
- 1 15.5 oz can chickpeas, drained, rinsed and drained again
- 12oz low FODMAP fusilli pasta, cooked until al dente and cooled slightly

Instructions:

1. Make the dressing by placing oil, vinegar, and mustard in a sealed jar and shaking. Season with salt and pepper.

2. Combine the warm pasta with the dressing and leave to cool for the flavors to amalgamate.

3. Add the feta, tomatoes, scallions, cucumbers, and peppers to the cooled pasta. Adjust the seasoning and chill before serving.

Nutrition Facts Per Serving

Calories 369, Total Fat 15g, Saturated Fat 1g, Total Carbs 49g, Net Carbs 46g, Sugar 3g, Fiber 3g, Protein 11g, Sodium 21mg

Penne with Gorgonzola & Walnuts

5 Ingredients

- 1 cup walnuts, chopped

- 1lb head radicchio, cut into 1-inch wide ribbons

- 6oz crumbled Gorgonzola or other mild blue cheese

- ½ cup flat-leaf Italian parsley, chopped

- Grated Pecorino Romano cheese, for serving

What you' ll need from the store cupboard:

- ¼ cup olive oil
- ¾ lb gluten-free penne rigate

- Salt and freshly ground black pepper

Instructions:

1. Toast the walnuts in a large skillet for 4 minutes, stirring frequently. Set aside.

2. Cook pasta until al dente according to package directions.

3. Heat the oil in a skillet and fry the radicchio for about 5 minutes. Season with salt and pepper.

4. Add gorgonzola and cook for 2 minutes. Add ½ cup of the pasta water and simmer for 3 minutes more.

5. Add the cooked pasta to skillet and toss to combine.

6. Add walnuts and parsley. e.

7. Serve in bowls and garnish with orange zest, if desired. Season with salt and pepper and offer more Pecorino Romano passed around.

Nutrition Facts Per Serving

Calories 656, Total Fat 46g, Saturated Fat 4g, Total Carbs 50g, Net Carbs 45g, Sugar 1g, Fiber 5g, Protein 18g, Sodium 1mg

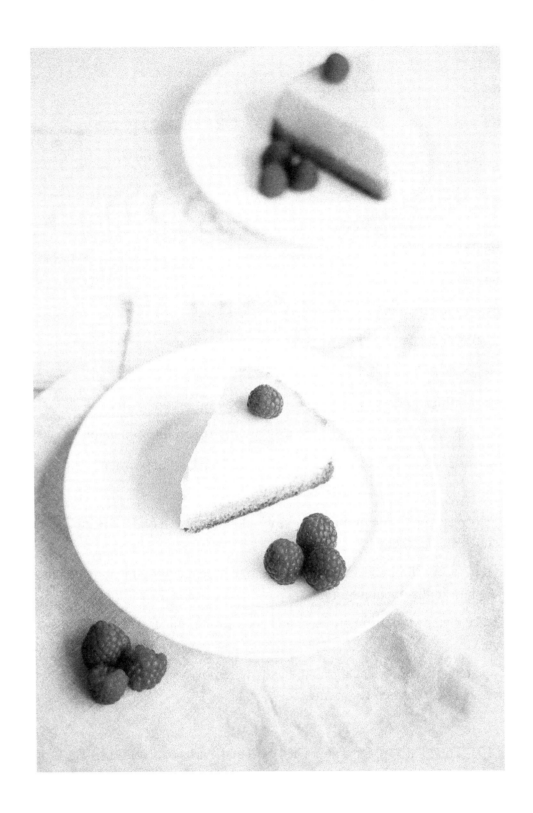

Dark Chocolate & Raspberry Pudding

Prep time: 5 minutes, cook time: 5 minutes; Serves 4

5 Ingredients

- ⅓ cup dark chocolate
- ¼ cup frozen raspberries
- 3 cup soy protein milk
- ⅓ cup fresh banana, sliced

What you' ll need from the store cupboard:

- 4 tbsp cornflour
- 1 tbsp cocoa powder
- 2 tbsp sugar

- ¼ tsp instant coffee
- ⅛ tsp ground cinnamon
- 1 tsp baking powder

Instructions:

1. Place chocolate and 1 cup of milk in a bowl and microwave on HIGH for 30 seconds or until chocolate has melted.

2. Put the sugar, cornflour, cocoa powder, instant coffee and ground cinnamon in a large bowl and whisk in the remaining milk.

3. Now place the bowl in the microwave and cook for 8 minutes and stir every two minutes.

5. Allow pudding to cool whisking periodically to remove any lumps. Decorate with raspberries and bananas before serving.

Nutrition Facts Per Serving

Calories 193, Total Fat 33g, Saturated Fat 19g, Total Carbs 6g, Net Carbs 5g, Protein 2g, Sugar 4g, Fiber 3g, Sodium 23mg

Cantaloupe Lime Popsicles

5 Ingredients

- 20oz ripe orange cantaloupe, cut into chunks

- 4 tsp freshly squeezed lime juice

What you' ll need from the store cupboard:

- ¾ cup water

- ⅓ cup sugar

Instructions:

1. Place the water and sugar in a small saucepan and simmer over a gentle heat, stirring all the time until the sugar has dissolved. Remove from the heat and allow to cool completely.

2. Put all the ingredients, including the sugar water in a blender and blitz until smooth.

3. Pour into ice pop molds and freeze until solid.

Nutrition Facts Per Serving

Calories 62, Total Fat 1g, Saturated Fat 0g, Total Carbs 16g, Net Carbs 15g, Sugar 15g, Fiber 1g, Protein 1g, Sodium 1mg

Bread and Butter Pudding

5 Ingredients

- 2 cups reduced-fat low FODMAP milk
- 1½ cup reduced-fat low FODMAP cream
- 10 slices gluten-free bread, crusts removed
- 1 cup blueberries
- 2 cup strawberries, hulled and sliced

What you' ll need from the store cupboard:

- 4 large eggs
- ¼ cup sugar
- ¼ cup maple syrup
- 1 tsp vanilla extract
- ½ tsp cinnamon

Instructions:

1. Grease a 2-inch deep, 7 by 12-inch baking dish.

2. Mix the eggs, sugar, vanilla, cinnamon, milk, and cream in a bowl.

3. Place the bread in the baking dish and pour over half of the custard. Sprinkle with half of the berries, then repeat.

4. Set aside

5. Bake in a preheated 350°F oven for 30 to 35 minutes.

6. Serve warm or cold.

Nutrition Facts Per Serving

Calories 260, Total Fat 12g, Saturated Fat 5g, Total Carbs 29g, Net Carbs 22g, Protein 10g, Sugar 12g, Fiber 3g, Sodium 200mg,

Coconut Popsicles

5 Ingredients

- 1 14oz can full-fat coconut milk

What you' ll need from the store cupboard:

- ¼ cup light corn syrup

Instructions:

1. Place syrup and coconut milk in a blender and blitz until smooth.

2. Pour mixture into 6 ice pop molds. Freeze overnight or until solid.

Nutrition Facts Per Serving

Calories 87, Total Fat 4g, Saturated Fat 0g, Total Carbs 12g, Net Carbs 12g, Sugar 5g, Fiber 0g, Protein 0g, Sodium 0mg

Rhubarb & Custard Cups

5 Ingredients

- 3 cup fresh rhubarb, chopped
- ¼ cup raspberries
- 4 cup low FODMAP milk
- 2 cups low gluten-free muesli
- 2 cup of low FODMAP milk

What you ' ll need from the store cupboard:

- 4 tbsp gluten-free custard powder
- 1½ tbsp sugar
- 1 tsp vanilla extract

Instructions:

1. Place the rhubarb and raspberries in a small saucepan and cover with warm water. Simmer for 10 minutes until rhubarb is tender.

2. Drain off liquid and mash the fruit.

3. Make custard with sugar according to directions on the packet. Add vanilla extract.

4. Layer the muesli, fruit, and custard into cups.

5. Serve immediately.

Nutrition Facts Per Serving

Calories 431, Total Fat 14g, Saturated Fat 3g, Total Carbs 71g, Net Carbs 66g, Sugar 26g, Fiber 5g, Protein 5g, Sodium 120mg

Fruit Salad

5 Ingredients

- 20 large fresh strawberries, cut into quarters

- ½ cup blueberries

- 1 large banana, sliced

- 1 large orange, diced

- 2 small kiwifruit, diced

Instructions:

1. Place all ingredients into a large bowl and mix well.

2. Divide the fruit salad into 4 serving dishes and serve immediately.

3. If you want to store the fruit salad in the refrigerator before serving, add a squirt of lemon juice to prevent bananas from browning.

Nutrition Facts Per Serving

Calories 86, Total Fat 1g, Saturated Fat 0g, Total Carbs 21g, Net Carbs 17g, Sugar 13g, Fiber 4g, Protein 2g, Sodium 0mg

Strawberry Frozen Yogurt

Prep time: 5 minutes, cook time: 0 minutes: Serves 4

5 Ingredients

- 1 cup strawberries, frozen
- 1 cup other low FODMAP fruit, chopped and frozen
- 1 cup plain thick lactose-free yogurt

What you' ll need from the store cupboard:

- 1 tbsp caster sugar/stevia powder/maple syrup/rice malt syrup
- 1 tsp vanilla essence

Instructions:

1. Place all ingredients into a food processor and blitz for a few seconds.

2. Don't over blend the yogurt as it will melt too much. Divide the yogurt

Nutrition Facts Per Serving

Calories 104, Total Fat 2g, Saturated Fat 1g, Total Carbs 14g, Net Carbs 10g, Sugar 14g, Fiber 4g, Protein 5g, Sodium 32mg

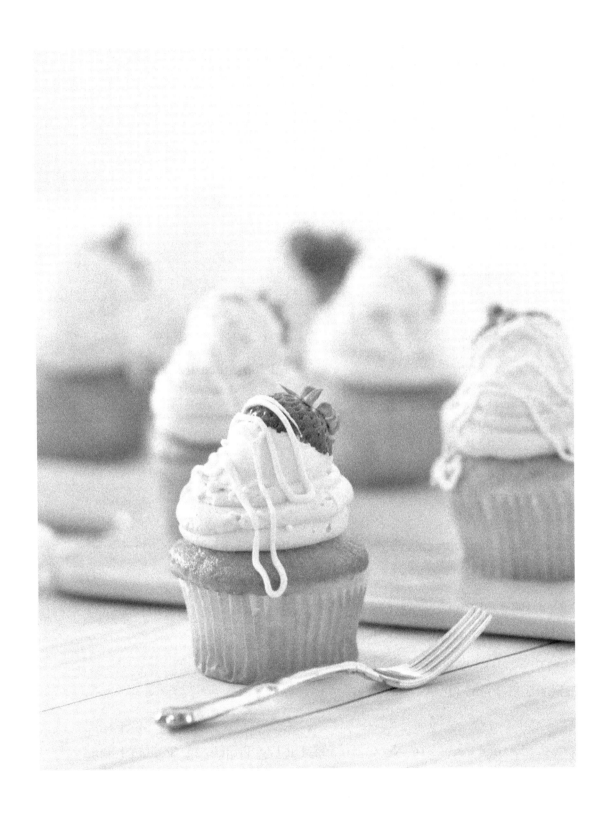

Almond Muffins with Blueberry

Prep time: 5 minutes, cook time: 30 minutes; Makes 12 muffins

5 Ingredients

- ½ cup almond meal

- ¾ cup almond milk

- ¾ cup blueberries

What you' ll need from the store cupboard:

- 1 tsp baking powder

- ½ cup caster sugar

- 1 tsp vanilla extract

- ⅔ cup vegetable oil

- 3 tbsp boiling water

- 2 cup gluten-free plain flour

- 1 tbsp chia seeds

Instructions:

1. Preheat your oven to 350°F.

2. Line a 12 hole muffin pan with paper liners.

2. Mix boiling water with chia seeds and stir carefully. Set it aside for 10 minutes.

3. Combine dry ingredients in a large bowl.

4. Add all remaining ingredients except blueberries.

5. Fold blueberries through the mixture.

7. Now, divide the mixture equally between 12 muffin cases.

8. Bake for 25-30 minutes.

Nutrition Facts Per Serving

Calories 285, Total Carbs 31g, Net Carbs 30g, Fat 17g, Protein 2g, Sodium 140mg

Berry & Yogurt Mini Pavlovas

Prep time: 2 hours, cook time: 60 minutes; Makes 8 mini pavlovas

5 Ingredients

- 1 cup strawberries
- 4 green kiwis
- 4 passion fruit
- 20 fresh blueberries
- ⅔ cup vanilla-flavored Greek yogurt

What you' ll need from the store cupboard:

- 3 egg whites
- ¾ cup confectioner's sugar
- 1 vanilla bean pod
- 2 tsp cornflour
- Pinch of salt

Instructions:

1. Preheat oven to 230°F.

2. Line an oven tray with baking parchment.

3. Take a large bowl and beat egg whites with salt until soft peaks begin to form.

4. Add the confectioner's sugar and continue beating with a spatula to make a glossy mixture.

5. Add cornflour and seeds from the vanilla bean pod.

6. Place the mixture into 8 even circles oven tray and bake for 2 hours until meringue turns crisp.

7. Combine fruit with yogurt.

8. Top each meringue with a dollop of fruity yogurt.

Nutrition Facts Per Serving

Calories 144, Total Fat 1g, Saturated Fat <1g, Total Carbs 31g, Net Carbs 27g, Sugar 29g, Fiber 4g, Protein 4g, Sodium 60mg,

Lemon Blueberry Pancake Traybake

Prep time: 10 minutes, cook time: 15 minutes; Serves 4

5 Ingredients

- 1 cup fresh blueberries
- 2 cup plus 2 tbsp low FODMAP gluten-free all-purpose flour
- 2 cup low FODMAP buttermilk
- 1 tsp lemon zest

What you' ll need from the store cupboard:

- ¼ cup sugar
- 2 tsp baking powder
- 1 tsp baking soda

- ½ tsp salt
- 2 large eggs
- 1 tsp vanilla extract

Instructions:

1. Preheat oven to 425°F.

2. Line a baking pan with parchment paper and coat with nonstick spray.

3. Combine the flour, sugar, baking powder, baking soda and salt in a large bowl.

4. In a separate bowl mix the buttermilk, eggs, lemon zest, and vanilla.

5. Add wet ingredients to dry ingredients and mix the batter well.

6. Pour batter into prepared tray and scatter with blueberries.

7. Bake for 15 minutes and serve immediately cut into 12 squares.

Nutrition Facts Per Serving

Calories 380, Total Fat 2g, Saturated Fat 0g, Total Carbs 81g, Net Carbs 78g, Sugar 18g, Fiber 3g, Protein 7g, Sodium 771mg,

Banana Bread

5 Ingredients

- 2 cup banana, firm, mashed
- ½ cup dairy-free spread
- 2 tbsp lemon juice

What you' ll need from the store cupboard:

- ½ cup brown sugar
- ¼ cup white sugar
- 2 large egg, lightly beaten)
- ½ tsp vanilla extract
- 1½ cup gluten-free all-purpose flour

- 1 tsp baking powder
- ½ tsp salt
- ½ tsp mixed spice
- 1 tsp baking soda

Instructions:

1. Preheat the oven to 350ºF.

2. Line and grease a loaf tin.

3. Cream the dairy-free spread and sugar together until fluffy.

4. Mix in eggs, mashed banana, lemon juice, and vanilla.

5. Add the flour, salt, mixed spice, and baking powder.

6. Transfer the mixture to the prepared tin and bake for 45 minutes.

7. Test the bread with a skewer to check if it is done before cooling on a wire tray.

Nutrition Facts Per Serving

Calories 239, Total Fat 9g, Saturated Fat 2g, Total Carbs 37g, Net Carbs 36g, Sugar 18g, Fiber 1g, Protein 3g, Sodium 120mg,

Lemon Cake

5 Ingredients

- ½ cup dairy-free spread, softened
- 6 tbsp lemon juice
- 3 tbsp lemon zest

What you' ll need from the store cupboard:

- 1 cup confectioners sugar
- 2 large egg
- ¾ cup gluten-free all-purpose flour

- ¾ cup white sugar
- 1 tsp baking powder
- ¼ tsp salt

Instructions:

1.Preheat oven to 350°F.

2. Grease a 12 inch by 8-inch tin.

3. Mix flour, sugar, salt, and softened dairy-free spread.

4. In a separate bowl whisk 2 tablespoons of lemon zest, 2 tablespoons of lemon juice and the eggs.

5. Pour the egg mixture into the dough and beat.

6. Pour batter into the prepared tin and bake for 20 to 25 minutes. Test with a skewer to check it is cooked through.

7. Make the icing by mixing the sugar with the remaining zest and juice. Pour over the cooled cake.

Nutrition Facts Per Serving

Calories 204, Total Fat 7.7g, Saturated Fat 1g, Total Carbs 32g, Net Carbs 32g, Sugar 24g, Fiber 0g, Protein 2g, Sodium 40mg,

Zucchini & Poppy Seed Muffins

Prep time: 10 minutes, cook time: 15 minutes; Makes 9 muffins

5 Ingredients

- 1 cup zucchini, grated with the excess water squeezed out
- 1 tbsp lemon zest
- 1 tbsp lemon juice
- 3 tsp poppy seeds

What you'll need from the store cupboard:

- 3/4 cup brown sugar
- 1/2 cup olive oil
- 1 tsp vanilla extract
- 1 large egg

- 1 cup gluten-free all-purpose flour
- ½ tsp salt
- 1 tsp baking powder
- ½ tsp baking soda

Instructions:

1. Preheat the oven to 350ºF.

2. Grease a muffin tin.

3. Mix sugar, olive oil, lemon zest, lemon juice, vanilla, and egg in a large bowl.

4. Add flour, salt, baking powder, and baking soda.

5. Fold through the poppy seeds and zucchini.

6. Spoon the batter into muffin tin.

7. Bake for 15 minutes until golden. Test with a skewer to make sure muffins are cooked.

Nutrition Facts Per Serving

Calories 256, Total Fat 14g, Saturated Fat 2g, Total Carbs 30g, Net Carbs 29g, Protein 2g, Sugar 17g, Fiber 1g, Sodium 120mg,

Cream Cheese Brownies

5 Ingredients

- ½ cup unsalted butter, at room temperature, cut into pieces
- ⅔ cup unsweetened chocolate, finely chopped
- 1 cup lactose-free cream cheese

What you' ll need from the store cupboard:

- ½ tsp baking powder
- ½ tsp salt
- 1¼ cup sugar
- 2 tsp vanilla extract

- 2 large eggs
- ⅔ cup plus 1 tbsp gluten-free all-purpose flour
- 2 tbsp sugar

Instructions:

1. Preheat oven to 325°F.

2. Grease and line an 8-inch square pan with non-stick spray.

3. Melt chocolate and butter in the microwave on LOW.

4. Combine the flour, baking powder and salt in a small bowl.

5. Stir sugar into the melted chocolate/butter mixture until well combined.

6. Beat in the eggs then stir in dry ingredients.

7. Spread batter into the tin.

8. Now mix the cream cheese, sugar, and flour in a small bowl.

6. Dollop the cream cheese mixture into the tin and swirl with a spatula.

7. Bake for about 30 to 35 minutes.

8. Cut into 25 brownies.

Nutrition Facts Per Serving

Calories 166, Total Fat 10g, Saturated Fat 2g, Total Carbs 19g, Net Carbs 18g, Sugar 13g, Fiber 1g, Protein 2g, Sodium 61mg,

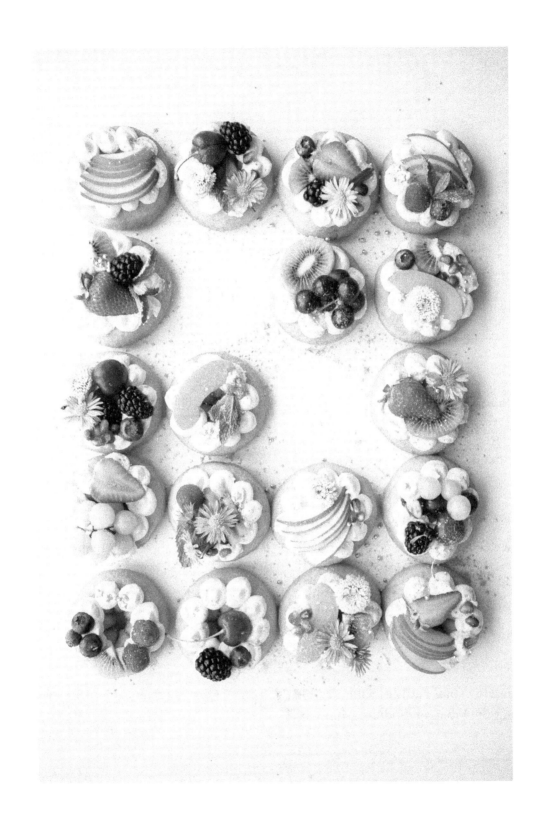

Peanut Energy Bars

Prep time: 60 minutes, cook time: 30minutes; Makes 12 bars

5 Ingredients

- ¼ cup dried cranberries
- ¼ cup dried banana
- ½ cup puffed brown rice
- 1 tbsp coconut flakes
- ½ cup almonds, lightly toasted

What you' ll need from the store cupboard:

- 1 cup rolled oats
- ½ cup quinoa flakes
- 1 tbsp chia seeds
- ½ cup maple syrup
- Cooking spray

Instructions:

1. Grease and line an 8-inch square tin.

2. Place the maple syrup and peanut butter in a saucepan and cook until melted.

3. Add remaining ingredients and stir well.

4. Transfer mixture to prepared tray and press down.

5. Refrigerate for one hour before slicing into 12 bars.

Nutrition Facts Per Serving

Calories 215, Total Fat 12g, Saturated Fat 2g, Total Carbs 19g, Net Carbs 15g, Protein 6g, Sugar 6g, Fiber 4g, Sodium 240 mg

Dark Chocolate & Cranberry Muesli Bars

5 Ingredients

- 1 cup dried shredded coconut
- 12 tbsp dried cranberries
- ½ cup dark chocolate chips
- 5 gluten-free weetabix, crumbled
- ½ cup dairy-free spread, melted

What you' ll need from the store cupboard:

- 1 tsp baking powder
- 1 cup gluten-free all-purpose flour
- 1 tbsp golden syrup

- 1 tbsp maple syrup
- 1 large egg
- 1 cup white sugar

Instructions:

1. Preheat the oven to 350ºF.

2. Grease a 9-inch square baking pan.

2. Combine all dry ingredients in a large bowl.

3. Whisk all wet ingredients in a separate bowl.

4. Add wet ingredients to dry ingredients and mix well.

5. Transfer mixture to baking pan and bake for 20 minutes.

6. Slice into bars while in the pan and still warm.

Nutrition Facts Per Serving

Calories 333, Total Fat 16g, Saturated Fat 7g, Total Carbs 49g, Net Carbs 46g, Sugar 32g, Fiber 3g, Protein 3g, Sodium 80mg,

Peanut Butter Cookies

Prep time: 10 minutes, cook time: 12 minutes; Serves 24

5 Ingredients

- 1½ cup peanut butter

What you' ll need from the store cupboard:

- 2 large eggs
- ¾ cup white sugar

Instructions:

1. Preheat the oven to 320°F.

2. Line two cookie trays with baking parchment.

3. Warm peanut butter in the microwave for 30 seconds on HIGH.

4. Mix all ingredients in a large bowl until well combined.

5. Drop tablespoon measures of cookie mixture trays.

6. Bake for 10 minutes. Two cookies equal one serving.

Nutrition Facts Per Serving

Calories 126, Total Fat 9g, Saturated Fat 2g, Total Carbs 4g, Net Carbs 1g, Sugar 8g, Fiber 1g, Protein 4g, Sodium 0mg,

Blueberry Crumble Slice

5 Ingredients

- 1 cup dairy-free spread, softened
- 3 cup blueberries

What you' ll need from the store cupboard:

- 1 cup sugar
- 3 tsp cornstarch
- 3 cups gluten-free self-raising flour
- 3 tsp baking powder
- ¼ tsp salt
- ½ tsp ground cinnamon
- 1 large egg, beaten

Instructions:

1. Preheat the oven to 350°F.

2. Grease an 8 by 12-inch baking pan.

3. Place ¾ cup of sugar, flour, salt, and ground cinnamon into a medium-sized bowl.

4. Mix the egg with dairy-free spread.

5. Add wet ingredients to dry ingredients.

6. Press mixture into prepared pan.

7. Top with blueberries.

8. In a small bowl mix cornstarch with the remaining ¼ cup of sugar.

9. Sprinkle over the blueberries. Bake for 30 minutes.

10. Slice into 15 pieces. Serve cold or warm with ice cream.

Nutrition Facts Per Serving

Calories 307, Total Fat 14g, Saturated Fat 2g, Total Carbs 42g, Net Carbs 41g, Sugar 18g, Fiber 1g, Protein 3g, Sodium 80mg,

One-Bowl Oatmeal Chocolate Chip Cookies

Prep time: 10 minutes, cook time: 12 minutes; Makes: 36 Cookies

5 Ingredients

- 1 cup unsalted dairy-free spread, melted
- 1 cup semisweet chocolate chips
- ½ cup raisins
- ⅔ cup walnuts, toasted, chopped

What you' ll need from the store cupboard:

- 1⅓ cup light brown sugar
- 2 teaspoons vanilla extract
- 1½ tsp cinnamon
- 2 large eggs

- 2½ cup old-fashioned rolled oats
- 1¼ cup gluten-free all-purpose flour
- 1 teaspoon baking soda
- ½ teaspoon salt

Instructions:

1. Preheat oven to 325°F.

2. Line two cookie trays with parchment paper.

3. Mix the melted spread and brown sugar until well blended.

4. Add vanilla, cinnamon, and eggs and mix well.

5. Stir in oats, flour, baking soda, and salt.

6. Finally stir in chocolate chips, nuts, and raisins.

7. Drop tablespoon measures of mixture onto the cookie sheets.

8. Bake for approximately 10 minutes or until golden brown.

Nutrition Facts Per Serving

Calories 206, Total Fat 9g, Saturated Fat 3g, Total Carbs 28g, Net Carbs 26g, Sugar 9g, Fiber 2g, Protein 3g, Sodium 92mg,

Milk Chocolate Chunk Cookies with Orange & Pecans

Prep time: 10 minutes, Chilling Time: 4 hours, cook time: 12 minutes; serves 24

5 Ingredients

- 1 cup unsalted dairy-free spread, at room temperature, cut into pieces

- 1 cup lightly toasted whole pecans, chopped

- 1 tbsp orange zest, finely grated

- ½ cup milk chocolate chunks

What you'll need from the store cupboard:

- 1 tsp baking soda

- 1 tsp salt

- 1 cup light brown sugar

- ½ cup sugar

- 2⅓ cup gluten-free all-purpose flour

- 2 tsp vanilla extract

- 2 large eggs, at room temperature

Instructions:

1. Combine flour, baking soda and salt in a large bowl.

2. Cream spread and sugar with an electric mixer until fluffy.

3. Beat in orange zest, vanilla, and eggs.

4. Stir in dry mixture ingredients.

5. Add chocolate and pecans and stir through the mixture.

6. Chill the mixture overnight in the refrigerator.

7. Roll golf-sized balls of dough and place on baking sheets lined with parchment paper.

8. Bake for around 12 minutes to make soft-baked cookies.

Nutrition Facts Per Serving

Calories 238, Total Fat 11g, Saturated Fat 1g, Total Carbs 33g, Net Carbs 31g, Sugar 14g, Fiber 2g, Protein 3g, Sodium 149mg,

Banana Maple Cookies

5 Ingredients

- 1 cup old-fashioned oats

- ½ cup gluten-free all-purpose flour

- ½ cup dried banana chips, chopped

- ½ cup unsweetened broad coconut chips or flakes

- 1 small very ripe banana fork mashed

What you' ll need from the store cupboard:

- 2 tbsp chia seeds

- 2 tbsp ground flax seeds

- 1 tsp cinnamon

- ½ tsp baking powder

- ¼ tsp salt

- ¼ cup maple syrup

- ¼ cup vegetable oil

- 1 tsp vanilla extract

Instructions:

1.Preheat oven to 325°F.

2. Line a baking pan with parchment paper.

3. Place the dry ingredients in a large bowl and mix well.

4. Mix mashed banana, maple syrup, oil and vanilla in a separate bowl.

5. Add wet ingredients to dry mixture and mix well.

6. Drop ¼ cup-sized cookies onto prepared tray. The mixture makes 10 cookies. Press the cookies down with your fingers.

7. Bake for 20 minutes.

Nutrition Facts Per Serving

Calories 178, Total Fat 10g, Saturated Fat 1g, Total Carbs 21g, Net Carbs 18g, Sugar 6g, Fiber 3g, Protein 2g, Sodium 77mg.

CPSIA information can be obtained
at www.ICGtesting.com
Printed in the USA
LVHW060141050222
710248LV00003B/49